Health Needs of the Elderly

Health Needs of The Elderly

Gill Garrett

SECOND EDITION

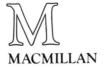

MACMILLAN

First published 1983
Reprinted (with corrections) 1984 (twice)
Second edition 1987
Reprinted 1988, 1990

Published by
MACMILLAN EDUCATION LTD
Houndmills, Basingstoke, Hampshire RG21 2XS
and London
Companies and representatives
throughout the world

Printed in Hong Kong

ISBN 0–333–44077–3

In memory of my parents . . . and for David and Rhiannon, past, present and future generations

Contents

Foreword to the series

This series of textbooks offers a fresh approach to the study of nursing. The aim is to give those beginning a career in nursing, and those already qualified, opportunities for reflection to broaden their approach to nursing education and to identify their own nursing values. The text includes material currently required by those preparing for qualification as a nurse and offers a basis for developing knowledge by individual studies. It should also assist qualified nurses returning to nursing, and those wishing to gain further insight into the nursing curriculum.

The authors of each book in the series are from widely differing nursing backgrounds, and, as experienced teachers of nursing or midwifery, they are well aware of the difficulties faced by nursing students searching for meaning from a mass of factual information. The nurse has to practise in the real world, and in reality nursing students need to learn to practise with confidence and understanding. The authors have therefore collaborated to illustrate this new perspective by making full use of individual nursing care plans to present the knowledge required by the nursing student in the most appropriate and relevant way. These textbooks can therefore be used in a wide variety of nursing programmes.

The practice of nursing — as a profession and as a career — and the education of the nurse to fulfil her role are affected by both national and international trends. The Nurses, Midwives and Health Visitors Act 1979 in the United Kingdom, the Treaty of Rome and the European Community nursing directives 1977, as well as the deliberations and publications of the International Council of Nurses and the World Health Organization, all make an impact upon the preparation and the practice of the nurse throughout the world.

Nursing values may not have changed over the past one hundred years, but society and the patterns of both life and care have changed, and are constantly changing. It is particularly important, therefore, to restate the essentials of nursing in the light of current practice and future trends.

Throughout this series the focus is on nursing and on the individual — the person requiring care and the person giving care — and emphasis is laid on the need for continuity between home and hospital care. *Neighbourhood Nursing — A Focus for Care*, the Report of the Community Nursing Review under the chairmanship of Julia Cumberlege (HMSO, 1986), has drawn attention to this need. The developing role of the nurse in primary care and in health education is reflected throughout this series. The authors place their emphasis on the whole person, and nursing care studies and care plans are used to promote understanding of the clinical, social, psychological and spiritual aspects of care for the individual.

Each book introduces the various aspects of the curriculum for general nursing: the special needs (1) of those requiring acute care; (2) of the elderly; (3) of children; (4) of the mentally ill; and (5) of the mentally handicapped. The latter category is dealt with by a new text in The Essentials of Nursing — edited by a well-known and respected nurse for the mentally handicapped and with contributors experienced in differing aspects of caring for people with mental handicap. The text on maternity and neonatal care, written by a midwifery teacher, provides the material for nursing students and would be helpful to those undertaking preparation for further health visiting education.

The authors wish to acknowledge their gratitude for the assistance they have received from members of the Editorial Board, and from all those who have contributed to their work — patients and their relatives, students, qualified nurses and colleagues — too numerous to mention by name. To all those nurse teachers who have read some of the texts, offering constructive criticism and comment from their special knowledge, we offer our grateful thanks. Last, we thank Elizabeth Horne for her contribution to the physiology material in the text, and Mary Waltham for her help with this second edition.

1987   Sheila Collins

Preface to the second edition

Since the first edition of *Health Needs of the Elderly* appeared in 1983 the demographic tide has continued to alter our population profile, and the need to reconsider our health approaches and to plan for future care becomes ever more urgent. In this second edition I have updated the original material and looked more to the future for our ageing society. Further to the comments of helpful colleagues and reviewers, I have included additional reading suggestions in each chapter, both to assist with the Pauses for Thought and to enable readers to follow up areas of personal interest.

1987

Gill Garrett

Acknowledgments

Many people have helped both directly and indirectly in the preparation of this book.

In the first group I should like to thank Mollie Clark for her criticism and advice on the text as a whole; Carole Clarke and Tina McKee for their comments on their specialist areas; and David Norfolk for all his encouragement and help with this second edition.

In the second my thanks are especially due to the very many elderly people with whom I have been privileged to work, in both hospitals and the community, over the past twenty years and from whom I have learned so much; and to the nursing students who, more recently, have helped me to learn further through their own learning.

My greatest debt of gratitude, however, is owed to the person who, more than anyone else, taught me through his own ageing experience of the needs of the elderly and who encouraged me to write about them—but who did not live to see the publication of the product of that encouragement—my father.

The author and publishers wish to thank the Trustees of the Copyright of the late Dylan Thomas and New Directions Publishing Corporation for permission to reproduce an extract from 'Do not go gentle into that good night', in *Collected Poems 1934–1952*, by Dylan Thomas. They also wish to acknowledge, with thanks, the following illustration sources, and to state that they have tried to clear copyright in all cases. Where they may have failed they will be pleased to make the necessary arrangements at the first opportunity.

Age Concern; Atlantech Medical; J. Brownhill; BBC Hulton Picture Library; J. Allan Cash Ltd; Central Office of Information/Department of Health and Social Security (Crown Copyright); Sally and Richard Greenhill; Robert Haines; Health Education Council (Christine Ottewill); Help the Aged; Philip Jackson; Terry Moore; *Nursing Times* (Alan Osborn); PACE Poulters; Press Association; WHO (T. Farkas, Philip Boucas and E. Mandelmann).

The remaining photographs were provided by the author.

A note on the series style

Throughout this book, in keeping with the other titles in this series, the term *nursing student* has been used to mean *both* student or pupil nurses *and* trained nurses who are undertaking post-basic training or who are keeping up to date with the recent literature. For clarity and consistency throughout the series the nurse is described as *she;* this is done without prejudice to men who are nurses or nursing students. Similarly, the patient is sometimes referred to as *he*, when the gender is not specifically mentioned.

Care plans, which are used throughout the books in this series, are indicated by a coloured corner flash to distinguish them from the rest of the text.

Part 1   Ageing

Chapter 1   The reality of ageing

Senescence, the genetically determined alteration in the structure and the functioning of an ageing organism, is a universal phenomenon occurring in all branches of the animal and plant kingdoms as it does in man. We are born, we grow through infancy and childhood, we develop to maturity; as the latter occurs over a period of time, again over a number of years, the processes of ageing render us 'old'. For all who survive assaults by illness or accident in earlier years, senescence is as much a fact of life as is its climax, death.

Not so senility, the state of functional disability consequent upon disease or trauma in the aged; this is sometimes referred to as secondary ageing in order to differentiate it from the natural processes of senescence, or primary ageing. An appreciation of the distinction between the two is vital for those in the caring professions; the elderly cannot be 'cured' of ageing, nor would the majority wish to be deprived of this normal, developmental progression in life. But the encouragement of positive health, the implementation of preventive measures to forestall disorders associated with ageing, and active rehabilitation should these occur are all integral parts of the work in which we are involved: the prevention of the secondary impinging on the primary.

Individuals age in different ways and at different rates, and react differently to the ageing experience. Emphasis in recent years has moved from a chronological definition of age to judging a person's physical and pyschological state in terms of his functional capacity, his ability to live actively and purposefully. Thus a person of 50 may be 'old', while another is 'young' well past the traditional three score years and ten.

Largely affected by retirement practices, however, our society has made the somewhat arbitrary decision that 'old age' begins at 60 or 65 and above this age researchers, government legislators and the public at large deem an individual elderly. Generalisations may have to be made — as they will be in the paragraphs that follow — but it is unwise to forget the facts behind the figures.

Life expectancy is affected by a variety of factors, ranging from the historical period in which one lives, family background, ethnic group and sex to lifestyle and contemporary technology. The great majority of individuals in Western society now live out their normal life span (women on average surviving the menfolk by some five years) and in the last 20 years — in keeping with trends throughout this century — the number of men and women past retirement age has risen by a third; they now form about 18% of the population as compared with 4.7% at the turn of the century.

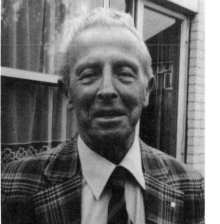

> **PAUSE FOR THOUGHT**
>
> What explanations can be given for:
>
> 1. The rising numbers of elderly in the population?
> 2. Their increased proportion within it?

Although improvements in the medical and public health services in general during the past century are often quoted as being instrumental in adding to the numbers of elderly within the population, they have been minimal in other than improving the quality of life and survival in a certain number of conditions. Since 1900 there has been very little improvement in life expectancy for people already in middle age — but a vast improvement for the newborn.

Victorian novels are full of accounts of little ones succumbing at an early age, 'taken by the angels' with a variety of conditions, infections featuring particularly high on the list. This century has witnessed a dramatic fall in maternal, infant and child mortality consequent as much upon improvements in general living standards, public hygiene and nutrition as upon advances in medical knowledge. This was complemented by a bulge in the birth rate at the begin-

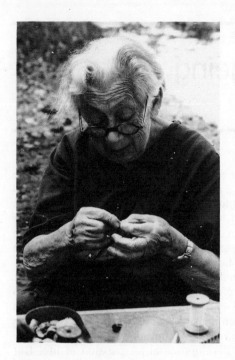

ning of the century and these two factors combine to explain the large numbers of elderly now found in the population.

The increased proportion of the elderly within the community has resulted from a falling fertility rate; with fewer babies born each year many countries in the Western world are moving with us towards zero population growth — and some have actually achieved this state. Yesterday's children have become the elderly of today with progressively fewer children and grandchildren of their own to even out the age balance within our society; for the section of the elderly for whom 'it is now normal for life to end as it began with a prolonged period of dependency', there are increasingly fewer carers to be dependent upon.[1]

Old age has been called 'the zenith of individuality'[2] and it would seem ironic that at this stage of life so often the 'elderly' are clumped together as a homogeneous whole. Since some 30 years of life may be included within this 'category', one obvious pitfall of which to beware is the assumption that the young old (the over 65s) and the older old (the over 75s and especially the over 85s) are one and the same in terms of lifestyle, outlook, needs and problems. The latter group are sometimes known as the 'vulnerable old' in that they are particularly at risk from physical, psychological and social trauma following the processes of ageing in our youth-orientated society; again, however, one must beware of generalisations, since many within this older age range often have quite exceptional mental and constitutional endowments and respond admirably to changing circumstances.

PAUSE FOR THOUGHT

Thomas Rees and Richard Smith both had their origins in a working-class background in a small town in the Midlands; the former is now 89, the latter 69. From your general knowledge of social history over the past hundred years can you describe the broad differences likely in their life experience?

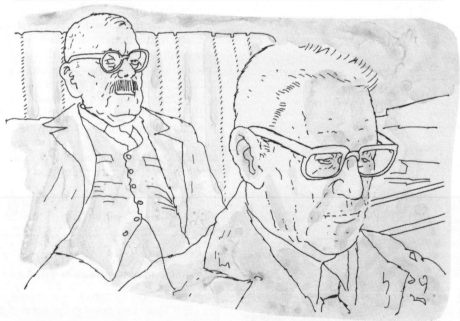

Perhaps your comparison of the two men's life experience demonstrated some of the broad differences given in Table 1.1.

Many other factors could have been included but those that have been outlined are sufficient to indicate the substantial diversities in life experience between two men of similar cultural and class backgrounds but of two different generations.

Given that one's experiences inevitably affect one's perception of life and response to it, especially when more individual features such as personality are additionally taken into account, it is obvious that the disparity between them will in no way be lessened simply because society, for convenience, deems them both 'elderly'. The failure to acknowledge essential differences and the assumption of blanket theories and policies thus reflect lack of insight and imagination in the onlooker or planner and can only act to the detriment of the older age groups.

Table 1.1   Comparison of two men's life experiences

	Thomas Rees	Richard Smith
Birth and childhood	Born in 1898, late Victorian era. Probably one of five or six children	Born in 1918 — average family size already falling
Formative years	Edwardian days of peace, prosperity and Empire. Clear definitions of social roles and class barriers	Turbulent times of the 1920s — days of social upheaval, greater personal opportunity
Education	Primary level — unlikely to have continued after age 13	Primary and secondary, possibility of grammar schooling
Great War	20-year-old fighting at the front	Not born until last year of war
Depression	Married man attempting to bring up a family	Still a child/teenager
Later employment	Low educational status likely to render manual/semi-skilled standing. May well have stayed in first occupation throughout working life	Employment and promotion prospects brighter, owing to better education. Working experience likely to include greater job mobility
Second World War	43 years old, serving in the Home Guard	Called up for active service
General adult lifestyle	Greater degree of continuity with previous generation. Probably carried out within fairly restricted locality	More material gains in working years, consumer durables, car, etc. Wider horizons in leisure pursuits
Retirement	Retired in 1961, unlikely to have worthwhile occupational pension. Of a work-orientated generation, adaptation may have been difficult	Retired 1983 — most likely has occupational pension (which may be index-linked) to supplement income. Probably better prepared for change in circumstances
Welfare State	Early years lived outside this. May still be reluctant to 'take from' the system	All his life lived within it — well used to manipulating the system
Losses	In childhood, perhaps siblings and one or both parents; then comrades in arms. In old age, spouse and friends; his own children may have predeceased him	Perhaps comrades in Second World War but losses minimal in comparison

References

1. Isaacs, B., Livingstone, M. and Neville, Y., *Survival of the Unfittest*, Routledge and Kegan Paul, p.8, 1972
2. Brown, M. (editor), *Readings in Gerontology*, Mosby, p.3, 1978

Further reading

Garrett, G., Ageing and individuals, *Nursing*, September, 1985, 1230

Stott, M., A personal experience of ageing, *Nursing*, September, 1985, 1203–1205

Blythe, R., *The View in Winter—Reflections on Old Age*, Allen Lane, Penguin Books, 1979

Chapter 2　　　The physiology of ageing

All cultures throughout the centuries have shown a fascination with the mysteries of the processes of ageing, some welcoming, some fearing (and anxious to retard!) their onset, depending on the view of the role and the relevance of the aged in the contemporary society. While the physical manifestations of ageing have always been apparent to the observer, however, any scientific study of the processes and the problems inherent within them has only been undertaken during the last half century. Gerontology is a multi-disciplinary subject, encompassing the study of the biological, psychological, sociological and economic aspects of later life.

Research during these 50 years has taught us much about the biological basis of ageing but it is generally agreed that there is no one cause of the phenomenon and that much further study will be required before a coherent, universally accepted theory is achieved. There is, however, acceptance of alteration at tissue, cellular and nuclear level, and a brief outline of some of the more common theories follows.

Biological clock theory

Champions of this theory propound the existence of an internal 'clock' governing the rate of cell activity and division and thus the timing of growth, decline and death. Its siting is open to conjecture; there may be an overall 'clock' in the brain, possibly in the hypothalamus, or each individual cell may have its own programmed timer.

Error accumulation theory

This proposes that environmental factors (such as radiation) cause genetic mutations which lead to ageing through faulty cell production and proliferation. Alex Comfort[1] has likened the two possible aspects of this theory to photographic reproduction; if a negative is scratched, all prints taken from it will be flawed; if the wrong chemicals are used in the process, although the negative may be perfect, the prints may be blurred.

Waste product accumulation theory

The concept here is that of gradual cellular decline as debris collects, possibly from the breakdown of intracellular membranes by chemicals known as 'free radicals'.

Chemical cross-linkage theory

This theory relates to the tissue level alteration seen in the elderly where collagen and elastin fibres in connective tissues 'knot' and fail to function properly. Some doubt has been expressed, however, as to whether this is an effect rather than a cause of ageing.

Auto-immune theory

The immune response is known to decline with ageing and it has been suggested that it may in itself be a causative factor in the process. Thymus mediated lymphocytes (i.e. those with their origin in the thymus gland) generally deal with any abnormal cells in the body by engulfing them and destroying them; their numbers are reduced with ageing, however, and the situation may then be aggravated by the production of new antigens by cell mutation.

For ease of description the main bodily systems of the ageing individual will be discussed separately but it must be remembered that 'the whole is greater than the sum of its parts' and that the functioning of each system is dependent upon that of the others. Note has already been made of the different rates at which people age; variation is also seen in the individual himself, as progression through the ageing experience does not occur at a constant rate, nor do all systems age simultaneously.

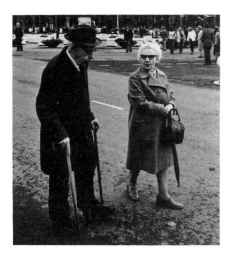

The musculo-skeletal system

Between the ages of 20 and 70 there is an average height reduction of two inches; the length of the long bones remains constant but there is shortening of the vertebrae with thinning of the inter-vertebral discs, reduction thus following from decrease in trunk length. Bone mass is reduced and muscle fibres atrophy, with fibrous tissue eventually replacing them; there is joint enlargement with fusion at the cartilage surfaces.

These changes ultimately lead to slower voluntary movement in the elderly and there may be a degree of muscle tremor at rest. The posture alters with slight backward tilt of the head and the varying degrees of flexion at the wrists, hips and knees leading to the development of a shuffling gait.

The excretory systems — skin and renal tract

(a) Skin

The wrinkling of the skin in ageing follows from the loss of tissue elasticity and the reduction in the amount of subcutaneous tissue. The epidermis thins and the surface blood vessels become more fragile; it is small haemorrhages from these that give rise to the very common purpura seen in the elderly. The sweat glands in the dermis atrophy with a reduction in perspiration and the nails thicken.

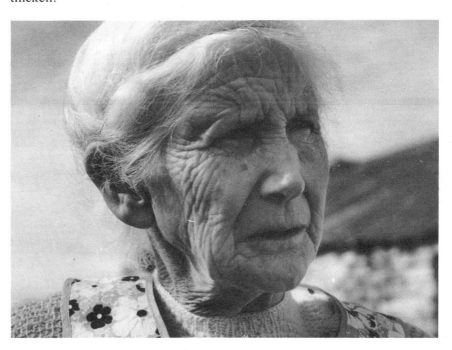

Greying of the hair is due to the loss of its pigment and the thinning seen in both sexes may be accompanied by balding in men. Bodily hair regresses everywhere except on the face; occasionally an increase here may be to the great embarrassment of the elderly woman.

(b) The renal tract

Nephrons are lost with ageing and the kidney size reduces accordingly. Blood flow to the kidneys drops by 53% and the glomerular filtration rate by 50% between the ages of 20 and 90. The frequency of micturition seen in the elderly is due to decreased bladder capacity and muscle weakness and is most noticeable at night, requiring more than three-quarters of older people to break their sleep. Physiological enlargement of the prostate gland in men may lead to urinary difficulties.

The gastro-intestinal tract

Dental loss is common in old age and gum recession occurs with advancing years. The flow of saliva is reduced and the gag reflex less efficient. Throughout the tract there is lessened motility with slower oesophageal and gastric emptying and a tendency to constipation because of lack of muscle tone; this may be exacerbated by a decreased secretion of mucus resulting in a less lubricated faecal mass.

Several factors combine to reduce absorption in the elderly and these include a change in gastric acid secretion, fewer cells on the absorbing surface of the small bowel and a reduced intestinal blood flow. As the liver becomes smaller there is delayed fat absorption and carbohydrate metabolism may be affected by decreased insulin production and utilisation (this is seen in 70% of the over 70s).

The cardio-vascular system

Anatomically the heart alters little with ageing other than becoming more darkly pigmented and showing some thickening of the valves. However, the contraction phase of the cardiac cycle is prolonged and the cardiac output drops by 40% between the ages of 25 and 65 (i.e. there is more energy expenditure for a less efficient result).

The blood vessels show reduced elasticity as collagen is laid down in their walls; to compensate for the increased peripheral resistance this produces, the blood pressure rises. A person's blood pressure will take longer to return to 'normal' after exercise or stress in later life than it did in his younger days.

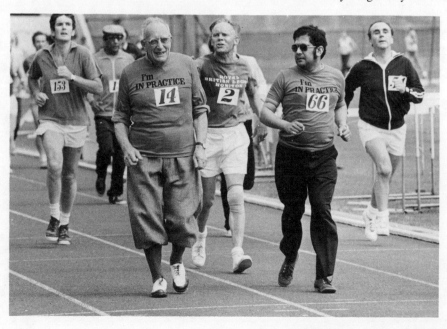

The respiratory system

As ageing progresses the lungs become less elastic and more rigid. There is a decrease in number but an increase in the size of the bronchioles and alveoli; consequently there is an enlargement of the wasteful 'dead space' (i.e. the space in the air passages not involved in gaseous exchange). Vital capacity is reduced by 25% in the elderly and by the age of 80 the pO_2 (arterial blood oxygen level) drops by 15%.

Weaker respiratory muscles may combine with decreased ciliary action and cough efficiency in the older person to render expectoration more difficult.

The nervous system

Brain weight decreases with age as neurons are lost. There is reduced conduction velocity along axons and thus response and reaction time is slower.

(a) The special senses

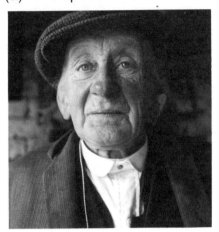

Generally in the older individual a higher threshold of stimulation is required for perception since sensory receptors are less efficient. For example, alteration in external temperature may not readily be appreciated nor prolonged pressure felt.

The number of taste-buds is significantly reduced during ageing, those sensitive to sweet and salt substances being affected earlier than those appreciating sour and bitter sensations. A reduced sense of smell may combine with this to cause diminished appetite.

Hearing acuity decreases with increased deposition of wax in the external auditory meatus, rigidity of the ossicles and atrophy of the eighth cranial nerve. Appreciation of the high-pitch frequencies is lost first but ultimately the older person may need to 'read' a situation by seeing the totality as well as hearing it.

Visual changes also occur with the pupils becoming smaller and less responsive to light. Accommodation is reduced as the lens becomes more opaque and the lens capsules less elastic; peripheral vision becomes narrower and colour perception is decreased.

The reproductive systems

The menopause marks the end of a woman's reproductive capacity. With the cessation of ovulation there is no progesterone output and the oestrogen level drops; the following changes are consequent upon this hormonal alteration.

The ovaries become thicker and smaller and the Fallopian tubes shorten; the uterus and cervix shrink. There is a loss of elastic tissue in the vaginal walls and the secretion of the mucosa reverts to an alkaline reaction. In the external genitalia there is a loss of subcutaneous fat and hair on the vulva, and a flattening of the labia, and the breasts become smaller.

Reproductive capacity is not lost by the older man although the number of viable spermatozoa produced decreases. His sexual arousal is slower with ageing and the number and force of ejaculations are reduced.

It must not be forgotten, however, that psychological factors play a crucial role in sexual relations and the changes outlined above in no way preclude the continuance of physical intimacy into extreme old age.

While discussion of pathological premature and accelerated ageing states are to be found in the medical textbooks, they are of limited interest to the nurse working with the elderly. The alterations to bodily structure and functioning described in the foregoing paragraphs are normal features occurring with the processes of ageing — they are not disease-related. An appreciation of them encourages an understanding of the adaptations in the activities of daily living which the older person may have to make — and the adaptations that may also be required of the nurse in her planning and implementation of care.

Reference

1. Comfort, A., *A Good Age,* Mitchell Beazley, p.111, 1977

Further reading

Comfort, A., *The Biology of Senescence*, 3rd edition, Churchill Livingstone, 1979

Bennett, G.C.J., The physiology of ageing. In Redfern, S. (editor), *Nursing Elderly People*, Chapter 3, Churchill Livingstone, 1986

Chapter 3 The psychology of ageing

'My memory is not what it used to be'; 'You can't teach an old dog new tricks' — how many comments are frequently made with the implication that mental deterioration in age is inevitable and inexorable, not only by the population at large but, as indicated by the first remark, reinforced by the elderly themselves? How true are these negative expectations of mental capabilities in later years?

Since life is lived within a social context and since behaviour is greatly affected by physical factors, it could be seen as somewhat artificial to consider the psychological aspects of ageing as distinct from these others. However, the physiological changes occurring with the ageing processes were outlined in the previous chapter and the sociological changes will be in the following; here we shall look at some of the findings in relation to personality, memory, learning, creativity and intelligence in older people, all of which indicate the effects of these variables upon the subjects in question.

Personality

In an interesting chapter in her book 'Growing Older — What You Need To Know About Ageing', Margaret Hellie Huyck[1] asks whether we age or grow older. In the absence of any gross pathological change, the personality remains constant into old age; 'for a growing person, time passing is parallel with the growth of self — you become ever more who you really are'. The inflexibility of which the elderly are sometimes accused generally results from physical or social restriction, not from personality change; it may simply represent caution in an unfamiliar situation.

Life calls for constant adaptation to change and there is, as Robert Butler puts it, 'a life-long identity crisis' as the person struggles to make sense of himself and his existence in an ever-changing world. Erikson,[2] the psychologist who identified for each stage of life a challenge to be met, described the challenge of old age as 'integrity versus despair'; in the face of many losses — of

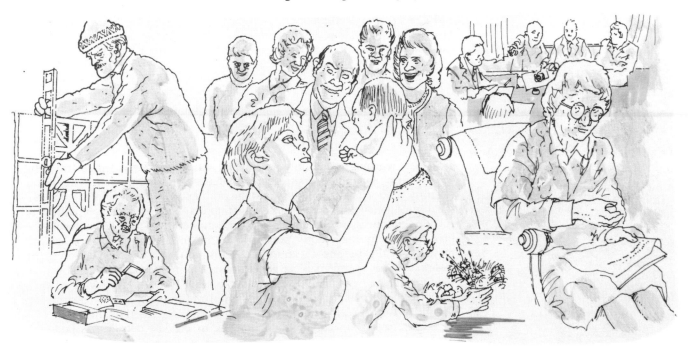

strength, health, perhaps family and friends — does the ageing person despair or transcend the crises? The vast majority of the elderly achieve 'integrity', employing different personality characteristics to do so; of the four personality types Bernice Neugarten[3] describes, only the 'disintegrated/disorganised' — a very small percentage of the elderly — show clear deterioration of functioning. The 'integrated' personality types reorganise their lives to cope with crises, sometimes focusing on other activities, sometimes voluntarily withdrawing into a rocking-chair attitude — still interested in the world but aloof from it; the 'defended' types, always having kept a tight rein on themselves, either keep busy and involved in order to feel worthwhile or shut out new situations to protect themselves from them; 'passive dependent' types react in the same way as they have throughout other hardships in life by seeking support and help from others.

As the personality remains constant in later years, so too does emotional capacity. Advancing age in no way diminishes the ability to feel joy or sorrow, pleasure or pain, love or rejection, contentment or anxiety. The overt response to the emotion may be less exuberant than in earlier years but this often belies the depth of feeling experienced by the older person, which should never be underestimated.

Memory

The memory loss of which the elderly may complain is of the short-term variety — where did they put the letter that came this morning? Who was it who telephoned yesterday? Long-term memory — often of completely inconsequential events, perhaps a picnic on the moors in 1926 when there was a torrential thunderstorm! — is preserved with remarkable clarity. Since the difficulty appears to be recall of a situation rather than recognition of it as familiar when reminded of it, it would appear that the problem is not one of coding and storing experiences for memory but of retrieving them when required. However, memory difficulties do not appear to be an inevitable feature of ageing; objective testing often shows little relationship between complaints of poor memory and actual performance. Where problems are found the subjects may be depressed or in poor general health; often strategies are developed to counteract the loss and it may only minimally interfere with daily living.

Where reminiscence is a common feature of an older person's conversation it should not be regarded as 'living in the past', as an unnecessary rehearsal of better days gone by. 'Life review' in the elderly as exemplified by reminiscence has been recognised as being of great value in integrating the diverse aspects of a life lived into a meaningful whole as its end is approached and as being essential for the maintenance of self-esteem, the ongoing achievement of which may be rendered more difficult in later life by illness or infirmity.

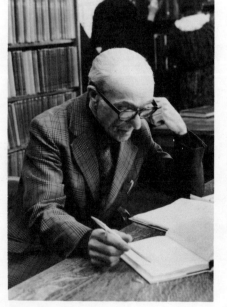

Learning

That new learning is certainly possible in old age is clearly demonstrated by those gaining Open University degrees when long past retirement! The slower reaction time seen in the elderly and the probable sensory deficits will necessitate employment of different teaching strategies — a slower pace, repetition of certain sequences, an emphasis on accuracy rather than speed — but where the task is seen by the elderly person to be meaningful (not some ridiculous psychological experiment!) and where he is motivated to achieve success, he will do so. Short-term goals are generally seen as more readily achievable than long-term ones, especially by the older elderly (presumably owing to their restricted time perspective); this has important implications when considering the setting of realistic objectives in care plans for elderly patients.

An interesting development in the UK in the last decade has been the growth of the University of the Third Age, which took its name from the

Université du Troisième Age, launched in France in 1972. Awarding no qualifications but dedicated to learning for its own sake, and acknowledging the priceless contribution older people can make to each other, it is open to the retired of any age. Members organise all kinds of educational and leisure activities based on the skills, knowledge and experience of their group. One of their stated aims is that 'by being seen to be involved in such challenging initiatives they will correct the public image of Britain's Third Age (i.e. retired) population . . . [who can] begin a time of creativity and fulfilment'.

Creativity

In addition to those artists who remained creative throughout old age — Rubinstein and Verdi into their 80s, Goethe and Picasso into their 90s—new talents have been developed and extended by others in later life; Grandma Moses, for example, staged her first exhibition when she was 80. On a more modest scale, the need within each one of us for a means of self-expression through which we can make a purposeful and valid contribution to the society in which we live — and to be valued for it — remains, however small the contribution or restricted the society.

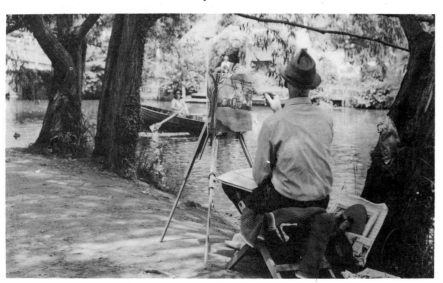

Intelligence

In recent years much research that had been undertaken into the effects of ageing on intelligence (and that had shown a decline in certain mental abilities) has been discredited. Questions have been raised concerning the validity of tests used, which initially were designed for young people; would not testing with problems specific to old age be more appropriate?

Also, to gain comparisons between a 20-year-old's mental ability and that of a 70-year-old shows nothing in terms of age differences generally. Where people of different ages undertake the same test (i.e. it is cross-sectional), differences in educational background, life experience, nutrition and health will inevitably affect the outcome. Only longitudinal studies (i.e. those on the same individual over a period of many years and therefore expensive and time consuming) could indicate specific differences with ageing — and then the results would be specific to that individual. The enormous variability between people is a vital consideration.

As with personality, mental ability, in healthy ageing, would appear to be preserved and constant; the bright 20-year-old, all things being equal, will be a bright 70-year-old; the not so bright 70-year-old would have been found in his youth to have had similar mental ability.

While the passing of laws of course does not ensure that the population obeys them, legislation has been passed against racism and sexism — but in the UK the far more subtle discrimination inherent in ageism has had no such consideration! We live in a youth orientated culture with emphasis upon production capacity and technological expertise and we retain a stereotyped idea of the elderly as those no longer active in this field. We exclude them from it because of economic factors (falling job numbers, rising unemployment) and the attitude that supports the 'prestige of youth'. To justify its exclusion of so large a sector of its community, society has to have a basis on which to do so; thus it excuses itself on 'their failing memories', 'their rigid attitudes', 'their difficulties learning new material'. This is the gist of the argument in Simone de Beauvoir's *The Coming of Age* (Penguin).

Of course many elderly are found who do exhibit the problems which might arise in old age, especially when physical health is poor. Much of the early gerontological research — from which some very negative conclusions were drawn — was carried out with the elderly in institutions who, removed from the stimulation of their own environments, no longer controlling their own destinies, showed marked mental decline. It takes time for society to unlearn what it has gathered — especially since the elderly themselves may anticipate such difficulties ('What can you expect at my age?') — rendering the ideas self-fulfilling prophecies.

Also, the media have of late woken up to their responsibility to inform the public of the plight of those elderly for whom problems exist. A number of extremely good programmes, discussions and articles have come out covering the considerable difficulties experienced by the elderly and their families which deprivation, depression and dementia may impose. Sadly, however, there has been little compensation with corresponding productions describing the positive manner in which the vast majority of the elderly manage their lives and day-to-day affairs; thus all the elderly are seen to be lonely, all the bereaved pathologically depressed and all the over 85s demented! Here the elderly themselves play a vital role in educating younger generations to accept as usual mental integrity in healthy old age; hopefully in years to come the comment 'Of course, she's marvellous for her age' will no longer be made — she will simply be accepted for the person she is, with the age factor of little significance.

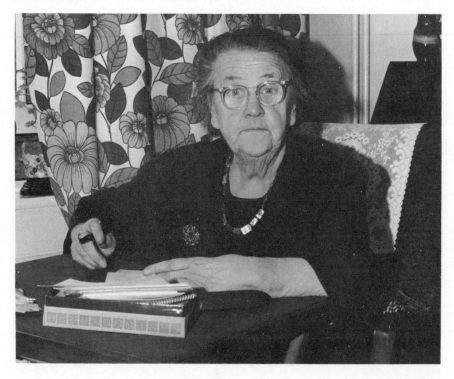

References

1. Huyck, M.A., *Growing Older — What You Need to Know about Ageing*, Prentice-Hall, 1974
2. Erikson, E., Growth and crises of the healthy personality, *Psychological Issues,* **1**, 1959
3. Neugarten, B., Grow old along with me! The best is yet to be, *Psychology Today,* **5,** No.7, 1971

Further reading

Midwinter, E., *Mutual Aid Universities — A Self-help Approach to the Education of Older People*, Croom Helm, 1983
Puner, M., *To the Good Long Life — What We Know about Growing Old,* Macmillan, 1979

Chapter 4   Sociological aspects of ageing

Since the period of 'old age' may span three decades, obviously the changes with which the ageing person must deal will vary from those occurring in his 60s — when his health, strength and companions may assist him in his adaptation — to those in his 90s — which he may be required to meet in less favourable circumstances, with poorer physical resources and fewer emotional supports.

The changes will not be described here as problems — though certainly to some that is what they may well be. They are perhaps better regarded as challenges to be met and dealt with. As indicated in the previous chapter, most of the elderly do achieve 'integrity'; even those who anticipate that such great social changes will prove insuperable ('I'd be lost without my work'; 'I depend so much on Jack, if it weren't for him I couldn't go on') generally cope with the situations when they do arise and, over a period of time, come to terms with them. It is the job of those in the caring professions to identify those for whom the challenges are problems — preferably before they have become so — in order to support them through the crises and to help them adapt their lifestyles thereafter; this is especially important where crises occur simultaneously, as they sometimes do with older people — for example, the death of a wife following closely on retirement — when coping mechanisms may well be stretched.

Retirement

Withdrawal from gainful employment is a relatively new phenomenon; in pre-industrial societies the older worker was obliged to continue at his job for as long as he possibly could. He only had his children or the 'Parish' to fall back on if illness or infirmity required him to give up; the former may or may not have been willing or able to support him, his fate with the latter was unenviable (*see* Part 2).

Now in the industrialised world there is an almost universal acceptance of the principle of retirement, although the age at which the worker must (in some cases) or can (in others) leave his employment varies widely — from 55 in Japan to 70 in the USA. Equally as varying are the attitudes of workers both to their occupations and to the necessity to give them up; studies have shown that,

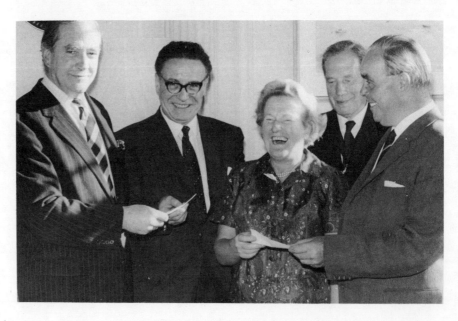

generally, the self-employed and the professionals are more satisfied with their jobs and happy to continue with them as long as they are able; those in less skilled, more routine jobs are frequently ready to withdraw from them at a much earlier stage, often before they are financially able to do so.

PAUSE FOR THOUGHT

Peter Townsend, the sociologist, has stated: 'To many working-class men retirement is a social disaster'. What reasons can you give for this?

For many working-class men retirement is often associated with four 'losses' which may explain the potentially disastrous outcome of the event for them. There is loss of:

1. Status and a role in society.
2. Companionship.
3. Income.
4. A meaningful lifestyle.

The Protestant work ethic is alive and well in Western society, upholding labour for its own sake as being the factor which, above all else, gives meaning to our existence. The problem that this poses to those rejected by the labour market as 'too old' has been appreciated for some time; now of course the difficulties are occurring in the younger age groups, for whom a recession means redundancy and unemployment in earlier years. Whether this will ultimately lead, along with the microchip revolution, to a reappraisal of society's values in relation to work remains to be seen.

Currently, however, one's status in society is still dependent upon one's involvement in a productive or supportive occupation. We are all guilty of asking, on first meeting someone, 'what he does'. How often the reply comes, 'Well, of course, I'm retired now, but I used to be . . .'; it is as if his self-esteem, his worthiness still depend upon his previous contribution in the working world and not on his present attributes as an individual.

For many men work is also a source of companionship and many out of work friendships have their basis in work relationships. After work and at the weekends, workers may meet in pub or club to play darts or skittles, cards or bowls. Where friendships can continue after retirement there may not be the same degree of involvement and financial constraints may make for problems, with difficulties in 'standing one's corner' at the bar perhaps or finding transport when a car has had to be given up.

Economists believe that between 65% and 80% of his previous income is necessary in retirement if the retiree's standard of living is to be maintained — and that does not take into account the effects of inflation. Patently, few people retiring today enjoy that level of income. Even where savings have prudently been made in earlier years they may rapidly be eroded in the first years of retirement, leaving the older elderly sorely disadvantaged.

Reduced finances may lead to many difficulties; in early retirement, social life and leisure pursuits may be limited — not only with friends but also with family. Townsend has written about the limitations to the 'gift relationship' hardship may impose — a couple may not accept an offer of a weekend with their children and their family, for example, because they cannot afford to entertain them in return. In later years, especially if the death of one of a couple has halved the income, reduced circumstances may lead to poor nutrition and the inability to maintain the home in a satisfactory, safe condition. With the present employment situation it is increasingly difficult for the retired worker to find work, full- or part-time, to supplement his income.

The loss of a meaningful lifestyle is tied up with the loss of status in society and follows from the scant recognition that is given to recreation and leisure activities; perhaps few working-class men have had the opportunity to develop these to any great degree in the first place. In very structured homes where male and female roles are clearly defined (as they are for many of today's retiring and elderly) involvement in home-making may be minimal; 'twice as much husband on half as much income' is for many women a true aphorism.

Most studies have to date concentrated on men in retirement as in previous years for most women paid employment outside the home was considered of secondary importance, and even for those who were employed elsewhere, as their role at home was seen to continue after cessation of employment the transition appeared easier for them. The anomaly in the situation was graphically described at the 1981 'Women in Later Life' conference organised by the British Society of Gerontology; women form the bulk of the population over 65 and 'the changing role of women calls into sharper question the earlier assumptions that women's experience of later life is marked by fewer tensions than is the case with men'.

For a decade now the importance of pre-retirement planning to facilitate the enormous change in lifestyle the challenge poses has been widely recognised. Jack Jones is quoted as having spoken of his belief that 'pre-retirement training should now become part of our collective bargaining in industry';[1] he sees employers having a duty to prepare their workers for retirement and to maintain links between former and present staff. Yet less than 6% of the 500 000 retiring in 1981 were thought to be receiving any organised assistance.

PAUSE FOR THOUGHT

As the Personnel Officer for a large brewery you are responsible for planning and organising the firm's Pre-Retirement Planning Course. Briefly (a) outline your course content and (b) indicate its timing in relation to retirement.

The course outlined below is one of two run by W.D. and H.O. Wills in Bristol and it covers all the subject areas which should appear in your plan — finances, health, recreational and educational opportunities. Interestingly, this course is residential, run at a conference centre owned by the company just outside the city; the participants are thus given the opportunity to take 'time out' away from the work situation to consider future plans in a relaxed setting. All staff from shop floor workers to management are included.

'A TIME TO LOOK FORWARD'

(Be sure that you have something better than good intentions to retire on!)

Tuesday

7.45 p.m.	Dinner
8.45 p.m.	Introduction
9.15 p.m.	'At the Crossroads' — discussion led by a recently retired couple

Wednesday

9.15 a.m.	The Imperial Tobacco Pension Fund
10.30 a.m.	Coffee
11.00 a.m.	Leisure Opportunities
1.00 p.m.	Lunch
2.15 p.m.	Budgeting and Investments
4.30 p.m.	Tea
5.00 p.m.	Health in Retirement
7.00 p.m.	Dinner
8.00 p.m.	State Pension and Benefits

Thursday

9.15 a.m.	Your Company Pension
10.30 a.m.	Coffee
11.00 a.m.	The Importance of Wise Eating
1.00 p.m.	Lunch
2.15 p.m.	Painting for Pleasure or Fishing For Fun
4.30 p.m.	Tea
5.00 p.m.	Income Tax
7.00 p.m.	Dinner
8.00 p.m.	Pensioners' Panel

Friday

9.15 a.m.	Your Future With Wills
10.00 a.m.	Coffee
10.30 a.m.	'The Way Ahead' — further discussion with recently retired couple
11.15 a.m.	Participants' Views and Comments
12.30 p.m.	Lunch

Since planning is called for over several years in preparation for retirement, a course offered in the last months of employment is obviously inadequate. Ideally information should be given regarding financial planning from the beginning of working life and the appropriate use of leisure encouraged from youth. The type of course described above may be offered some two to three years before retirement, with intermittent follow-up sessions, perhaps in social settings, until the time of leaving. Many of the larger firms are now organising post-retirement meetings and some utilise recently retired personnel to maintain contact with older retired workers.

Family changes

To many elderly the family unit retains its central position and — contrary to popular belief — there is still much contact between generations within families, although this may be less frequent and intimate than in previous years (*see* Part 2). But, as gender roles are changing, so are roles within the wider family and adaptation may be called for on the part of older people.

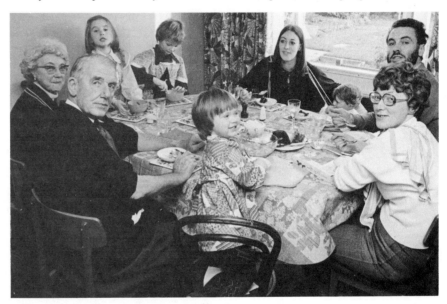

As their children have grown up and begun families of their own, parents will have been required to view them in a new light — as equals rather than as dependants in the family situation; rivalries may be engendered by this but they are generally worked out satisfactorily and a balance achieved. The changing emphasis in society on women as workers as well as carers and on men as carers as well as workers may be difficult for the older generation to appreciate, however, and may be the source of some contention. Older women who have lived primarily as wives and mothers and men as protectors and providers may feel that all those years now have little value in the eyes of their offspring.

The nature of grandparenting has also changed in recent years, especially where there is a highly mobile population. Although much valuing their contact with their grandchildren, the elderly generally find that they are no longer expected as in previous years to be intimately involved in their upbringing. Charlotte Eliopoulos[2] points out that this is by no means a negative aspect; in addition to the younger adults having more definite control over their lives, 'older adults often enjoy the independence and freedom from responsibility that nuclear family life offers'.

It is important, however, to remember that in some social groupings elderly people often continue to play a very active caring role in family situations. In a study in Cumbria in 1978 almost two-thirds of the elderly people who had children were found to be actively engaged in babysitting, shopping, lending money or caring for and cooking for school-aged children, often freeing mothers to undertake paid work.[3] In the wider 'family' sense elderly people are often the source of help to other elderly people to whom they are close; one study found that 30% of the disabled elderly were receiving help from such a source.[4]

For most of the elderly, the biggest change in lifestyle is inevitably brought about by the death of a partner — be it a marriage partner, a long time friend or a sibling. A man left alone after a lifetime of care from a female partner, in addition to his grief, has to contend with the practicalities of everyday living, cooking, washing and housework. For a woman who has had little dealings with the business aspects of life, there may be financial difficulties and she has little chance of finding work after a lifetime in the home. We still live in a couple-orientated society and social involvement may be limited when half of one becomes a single within it. Sexual needs may remain unfulfilled in the single state; sadly, the freedoms accorded to the younger generations are not as yet accepted for the elderly or sometimes — owing to earlier upbringing and beliefs — by the elderly themselves. The ongoing need for affection, physical closeness and warmth in no way abates in later years but the means for its fulfilment often do.

While retirement and family changes are for the most part encountered and dealt with in early old age, the situations leading to loneliness and role reversal generally occur in later years and may therefore be more difficult challenges to meet.

Loneliness

It is most important that a distinction be made between loneliness and aloneness; the latter is often enjoyed by the elderly for periods of time, as solitude gives the chance to reflect, to recollect one's energies. Loneliness, however, means isolation even in company; it is notable that many of the elderly who

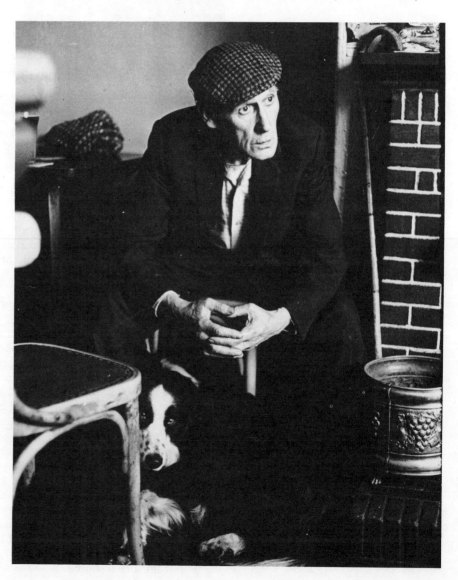

complain of loneliness are found in residential care or in hospital, where they are in no way alone.

There are many possible reasons for loneliness: geographical (rural districts having poor transport services, urban ones having inhibiting crime rates), physical (sensory losses leading to difficulties in communication or perhaps incontinence leading to social withdrawal) as well as emotional (the loss of loved ones to time and death at the end of a long life). The underlying factor in this last situation of course is not remediable — many of the older elderly face it, however, with equanimity; that the others are, but are allowed by our society to persist and thus to limit socialisation in later life, says much about our attitudes and priorities.

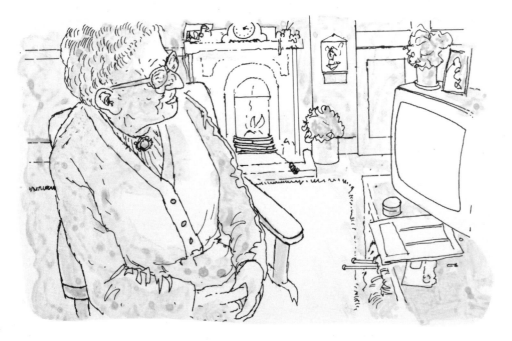

Role reversal

For those older elderly for whom later years are dogged by declining health and consequent dependency, upon either their families or other agencies, the psychological distress brought about by the situation may be far more difficult to bear than the physical incapacity suffered. How frequently the phrase 'I don't want to be a burden!' is repeated in ageing — and even in earlier life — indicating the fear that this is how one's life will, somehow ignobly, end.

In their earlier years, as parents, the elderly cared for their offspring, sheltering and nurturing them; when the young grew to independence, the balance mentioned above was attained and the generations viewed one another as equals. Role reversal may occur, with the elderly parents becoming dependent upon their adult children as illness or advanced age overtakes them. Equally the elderly may in younger years have played supportive roles in a wider society which is now required to support them. Where dependency sits uneasily upon the elderly there may be evidence of stubbornness and an unrealistic attitude to the situation; where the new carers have not come to terms with it, there may be resultant resentment and depression.

If the sociological aspects of ageing present the elderly with challenges to be met, they do so equally to society as a whole. The 'disengagement theory' of Cumming and Henry,[5] popular in the 1950s, which postulated that the gradual withdrawal of the elderly and the world from each other was essential for 'successful' ageing, has been largely discredited; it could have been seen as condoning society's tardiness in catering for the older age groups. The 'activity theory' of Havighurst, Maddox and Palmore, which states that the elderly need to maintain as much as possible their former levels of involvement in family, social and civic activities, is much more widely held; it needs, however, to be acted upon in terms of social policy to ensure that as many of the elderly as possible are able to do so.

References

1. Stott, M., *Ageing for Beginners*, Blackwell, p.77, 1981
2. Eliopoulos, C., *Geriatric Nursing*, Harper and Row, p.32, 1979
3. Butcher, H. and Crosbie, D., *Pensioned Off*, University of York Cumbria Development Project, 1978
4. Green, S., Creese, X. and Kaufert, J., Social support and government policy on services for the elderly, *Social Policy and Administration*, **13**, 1979, 210–218
5. Cummings, E. and Henry, W., *Growing Old*, Basic Books, 1961

Further reading

Tinker, A., *The Elderly in Modern Society*, Longmans, 1984; especially Chapter 11, The contribution of the elderly

Silver threads — preparing and planning for old age, *British Journal of Geriatric Nursing*, **4**, No. 1, 1984, 3–7

Chapter 5   Demographic and economic aspects of ageing

The first chapters of this book have considered ageing from a broadly individual perspective, physically, psychologically and sociologically. In this chapter a more statistical viewpoint is taken in looking at the actual numbers and situation of elderly people in Great Britain today. Mention has already been made of the vital need to see elderly people as individuals and to avoid blanket theories, but to enable rational forward projection and planning to take place it is also essential to comprehend these demographic and economic aspects of our ageing population.

How many elderly people?

PAUSE FOR THOUGHT

Study Figure 5.1 and Table 5.1 From the information contained within them, describe the demographic changes occurring in the 1970s, 1980s and 1990s for:

(a) the 60/65–74-year-olds
(b) the 75–84-year-olds
(c) the over-85-year-olds

During the 1970s the number in the first age group increased by 0.2 million (out of a total increase in the elderly of 0.9 million). Throughout the 1980s the number of people of this age group is expected to decrease slightly, with a more pronounced drop in the following decade.

Table 5.1   The elderly population of Great Britain by broad age-groups. Source: Office of Population Censuses and Surveys, Census Guide 1, Britain's Elderly Population, 1981 Census

Census data					Projections	
	1951	1961	1971	1981	1991	2001
Number by age (millions)						
60–64 Women	1.3	1.5	1.7	1.5	1.5	1.4
65–74 Women	2.1	2.3	2.7	2.8	2.8	2.5
Men	1.5	1.6	1.9	2.2	2.2	2.1
Persons	3.6	3.9	4.6	5.0	5.0	4.6
75–84 Women	0.9	1.2	1.4	1.7	1.9	1.9
Men	0.6	0.7	0.7	0.9	1.1	1.1
Persons	1.5	1.8	2.1	2.6	3.0	3.0
85 and over Women	0.2	0.2	0.3	0.4	0.6	0.8
Men	0.1	0.1	0.1	0.1	0.2	0.3
Persons	0.2	0.3	0.5	0.6	0.8	1.0
Total numbers (millions)						
60/65 and over	6.7	7.6	8.8	9.7	10.3	10.1
75 and over	1.7	2.3	2.5	3.1	3.8	4.1
85 and over	0.2	0.3	0.5	0.6	0.8	1.0
Population, all ages (millions)	48.9	51.3	54.0	54.3	55.4	56.4

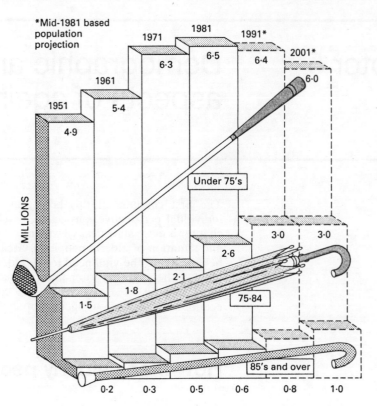

Figure 5.1 *Numbers of the elderly by broad age groups, Great Britain, 1951–2001. Source: Office of Population Censuses and Surveys, Census Guide 1, Britain's Elderly Population, 1981 Census*

The 75–84-year-old age group increased more substantially in the 1970s — there were some 0.5 million more people of this age by the 1981 census than there had been in 1971. During the 1980s the rate of increase is expected to slacken somewhat, and then numbers will remain static throughout the 1990s.

However, the most dramatic demographic changes occur in the over-85-year-old age group. The 1970s saw an increase of 0.1 million, comparable in fact when expressed as a percentage with the increase in the 75–84-year-old range. During the 1980s, though, far from slackening off, as is the latter, the rate of increase is accelerating rapidly, and numbers will continue to rise during the 1990s, with an expected 1.0 million of the population having achieved this age by 2001. Although the percentage increases may seem small, it is highly significant that in 1971 5.71% of the elderly were over 85; by 1981 this had risen to 6.2% and by 1991 it is expected to be 7.8%. When speaking of our 'ageing population', it is important to remember that its most obvious feature is its own ageing age structure.

When looking at the balance of men and women in the elderly age groups, striking differences are immediately apparent. The statistics show that on reaching pensionable age only one-third of the population is male. However, this finding is somewhat distorted by the present earlier retirement age for women; if this is allowed for, the numbers are more nearly equal. By the time we reach the 75–84-year-old age group, though, there are actually two women for every man, and beyond the age of 85 women outnumber men by four to one. Thus, in the ageing age structure, an increasing majority are women.

What are the implications of this gender imbalance? In terms of marital status, in 1980 49% of women in the over 75 age group were widows, with 35% still married, whereas 17% of men were widowers and 75% were still married. Eleven per cent of all elderly women had never married, but in the over 85 age group this rose to 16% (reflecting the effects of the First World War on marriage patterns). Two per cent of the elderly overall were divorced. Figure 5.2 illustrates the projected situation in 2001. Of the 52% of the over 65s who were living with a spouse in 1980–1981 the majority were men.[1] The majority of elderly women live alone and may have done so for a long time; also, because of the gender imbalance, many more elderly women are in institutional care than are men.

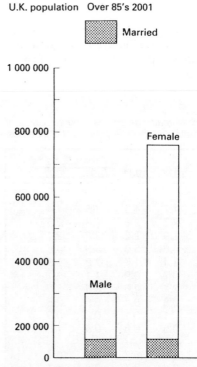

Figure 5.2 *Projected population in 2001– marital status. Source: Office of Population Censuses and Surveys, Census Guide 1,* Britain's Elderly Population, 1981 Census

In total some 3% of the elderly live in a communal establishment such as a residential or a nursing home — only 1% of the under 75s but 19% of the over 85s being in such environments. The number of elderly people living alone has doubled since 1961 and now almost 25% of all households contain only elderly people; this is a very significant percentage, since the people in such situations may be very vulnerable to financial and domestic difficulties.

Where are they now?

PAUSE FOR THOUGHT

From your general knowledge of change over the past 60 years can you describe how the geographical distribution of elderly people may have altered during that time?

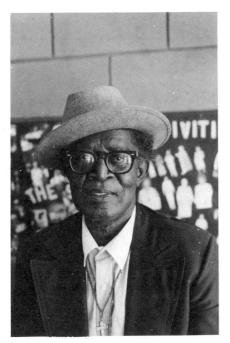

Sixty years ago many rural areas contained a high proportion of older people, with younger people moving to the industrial areas for employment. Those younger people have now aged, however, giving an older profile to inner city areas, and — other than in districts such as Central Wales and the Borders — the more rural areas have now regained a younger population, with families moving out of urban living. Many of the post-war city rebuilding schemes which saw an influx of young and middle aged couples in the 1950s are now housing those same couples in their later years. A significant rise in the number of elderly people from ethnic minorities has also been apparent (there are, for example, now some 50 000 elderly people of New Commonwealth and Pakistani origin in the UK) and the great majority are living in inner city areas.

Retirement to seaside resorts has long been a feature of British life, and from the 1920s onwards towns such as Eastbourne and Bournemouth experienced a steady rise in their elderly populations which has only slackened off over the last decade. The effect of this has been to leave towns such as Worthing with a population of whom 35% are over retirement age (the national average being 18%). On the other hand, new towns have a much lower than average proportion of elderly people in the population — for example, Redditch has only 11% and Cumbernauld 9%.

It would seem that elderly people are now a more 'static' population than their younger counterparts. At the 1981 census about 5% of those past retirement age had moved in the previous year, 9% of the rest of the population having done so. The vast majority of those changing homes had made only very local moves (within 30 miles).

How well off are they?

On the conventional definition of poverty (i.e. those at Supplementary Benefit level), 2.5 million of the elderly are below the poverty line, with a further 3.7 million being on the margin. Together these figures encompass 66% of the elderly population. In his book *Poverty in the United Kingdom* (Penguin), Peter Townsend describes the dual causation of this as being the low life-long class status of many elderly people and society's imposition of an 'underclass' status on them now. Certainly, because of discriminatory employment and welfare legislation in the past, compounded perhaps by long periods out of the work force to undertake caring duties within the family, many elderly women are facing severe economic difficulties now. Alex Comfort writes: 'Adequate money is the most important single thing which separates a good from a bad old age . . . enough money is the thing older people need most.'[2] Whether or not one totally agrees with the sentiment of this statement, there can be little argument that the quality of life in old age depends to a large extent on the adequacy of an elderly person's income to meet his individual needs. It is interesting to recall the words of Beveridge, an architect of our welfare state: 'Any plan of Social Security worth its name means providing as an essential part of that plan a pension on retirement from work which is enough for subsistence.'[3] Good health, both physical and mental, demands the appropriate resources for shelter, heating, food, clothing and social activity, and in our present society many elderly people existing solely on a retirement pension simply do not possess these. It is important to remember that not all our elderly population receive a pension in the first place — some 17% of Afro-Caribbean elderly in Britain do not, nor do 54% of the Asian elderly here. Indeed 6% of the indigenous population are not entitled to a retirement pension.

Table 5.2 *Selected amenities for 'elderly only' households, Great Britain, 1981. Source: Office of Population Censuses and Surveys, Census Guide 1, Britain's Elderly Population, 1981 Census*

Amenity	All households	Percentages of households			
		Elderly only households			
		Total	Lone man	Lone woman	Two or more pensioners
Lacking bath	1.9	4.1	6.9	4.7	2.7
Lacking WC	2.7	5.0	8.0	5.2	3.9
One or more persons per room	4.3*	5.2	6.1	4.3	6.0

*Over 1 person per room.

This financial discomfiture is reflected in the housing and amenities situation of many elderly people. The reader will find a more comprehensive discussion of housing deficiencies in the section on 'A suitable environment' in Chapter 8, but the details given in Table 5.2 outline the scale of the problem. Ready access to reasonable transport facilities may also be prejudiced where finances are severely limited; for many elderly people a car would represent the most useful form of transport, but only 27% of elderly households have the use of one, as compared with 61% of all households.

The number of elderly people in paid employment, working to supplement their pensions and benefits, has dropped over the last 20 years, as Table 5.3 below indicates. Of those in employment at the time of the 1981 census, 66% had part-time work only; this may have reflected their personal desires or may be indicative of the situation in the job market generally. Because of the current level of unemployment among younger people, older workers who wish to continue at their occupations, or to find new ones, and who could usefully do so, may now meet considerable resistance from prospective employers and people generally. Earnings limits imposed by the Government also militate against elderly people working past pensionable age.

Table 5.3 *Elderly people in paid employment (%)*

Category	1961	1971	1981
Women over 60	10	12	8
Men over 65	25	19	10

References

1. Central Statistical Office, *Social Trends,* **13**, H.M.S.O., London, 1982.
2. Comfort, A., *A Good Age,* Mitchell Beazley, London, 1977.
3. H.M.S.O., Cmnd 6404, para.239, p.92, 1942.

Part 2 Approaches to Ageing: Evolution of Care

Chapter 6 Family and welfare approach

'I'd rather die than go to the workhouse'; although it is now more than 50 years since the passing of the Act abolishing Poor Law Institutions, the disgrace and degradation associated with 'the workhouse' is vividly recalled by the elderly to this day. The fact that, on the demise of the old system, many of the redundant buildings were pressed into service as geriatric units has reinforced for these elderly the impression that the institution has simply changed its name; its grim physical exterior and the persistence of the old reputation for inhumanity and harshness have frequently been detrimental to the attempts at increasing awareness of the current emphasis of work with older patients — individualised care, progressive treatment and active rehabilitation.

Some understanding of the evolution of the provision of care for the elderly would seem to be important to the nursing student dealing with older patients if possible fears and anxieties are to be allayed.

For more than three centuries after the Poor Law Act was passed in 1601 the needy elderly came under the same classification as the sick and destitute of any other age group – 'the impotent poor'. Their support was initially the responsibility of the parish in which they resided; under Gilbert's Act of 1782, parishes were allowed in addition to combine into Unions to establish reformed work-houses in which custodial-type care could be given. The control of these workhouses passed from the parishes to central government under the Poor Law Amendment Act of 1843 and 'out relief' was virtually discontinued; the destitute were obliged to enter institutions. Conditions within them were well documented both in current literature (such as Dickens's *Hard Times*) and in contemporary sociological reviews; as indicated above, they were personally experienced by a few of today's older elderly and well known to the others by word-of-mouth accounts.

The Royal Commission led by Lloyd George in 1905 marked the beginnings of the Welfare State as we know it today; even before it reported in 1909, the budget of the previous year had decreed the payment of a weekly pension of 5/- (25p) to those over the age of 70. This was a non-contributory benefit; it was followed three years later by the National Insurance Act instituting a contributory scheme to cover periods of ill-health and to provide free medical attention. Those not covered by the scheme (i.e. those not in paid employment) were still required to pay for treatment until after the Second World War; in 1947 a consultation with the doctor cost 1s. (5p) and a home visit 1s. 6d. (7½p). The

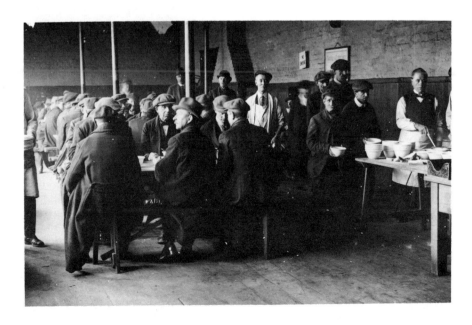

final nail was only put into the Poor Law coffin in 1948 with the inception of the National Health Service and the passage of the National Assistance Act, unifying retirement pensions with other benefits and, in Part III, requiring local authorities to provide accommodation for the aged and infirm.

Family care

Contrary to popular belief, in pre-industrial British society the strong arms of the extended family network did not of necessity encompass the aged when they became infirm or simply too old to work. Peter Laslett,[1] writing about the management of our present situation, states that it 'calls for invention rather than imitation'; the past which we erroneously feel that we should imitate saw far fewer of the population achieving old age in the first place and, for those who did, their support by their offspring was dependent more upon their mutual affection than upon external social pressures.

> PAUSE FOR THOUGHT
>
> Despite this, it is probably true to say that in the time of extended families the elderly that there were, were more likely to be surrounded by relations with more frequent access to help from them.
>
> In terms of looking after their own elderly within the family environment, it may now be more difficult for relatives. What explanations could be given for this in the light of social and demographic changes in recent years?

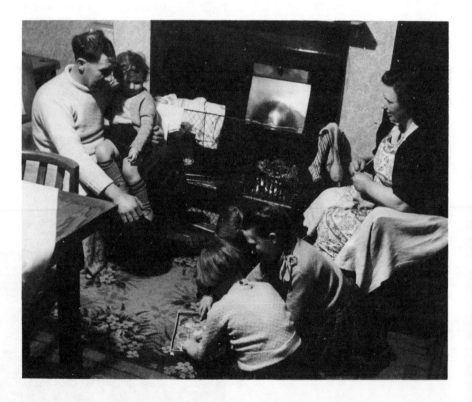

The family context in which today's elderly grew up differed markedly from that in which they see their children and their children's children now living. Marriage now occurs earlier and the nuclear family has replaced the extended; two- rather than three-generational households are the norm, with housing generally being of a smaller design.

Moral values and social mores have altered vastly in the last half century and ways of child rearing with them; tremendous tensions can result in families of three generations, the older two disagreeing on the needs and responsibilities of the youngest and the freedoms afforded to it. Alex Comfort[2] has pointed out how people today appear to be in a stage of transition from 'family orientation' to 'peer orientation', a situation relatively foreign to the elderly. He also discusses the trend to second marriages following divorce as a stumbling block in the path of inter-generational unity.

Earlier generations generally sought employment in local trades and industries, sometimes remaining at their original job for the whole of their working lifetime. Mobility is now a factor inherent in continuing employment for most people and may require the offspring of elderly parents to live many miles from the parental home, in another city or — not infrequently — in another country.

However, perhaps the greatest change affecting the family and its provision for its elderly has been the altered role of women in society; traditionally the carers for and supporters of offspring and other dependants, they have now to combine this role with the demands made upon them by social and professional attainments of recent years. The majority are in paid employment and many are pursuing ongoing careers; although still inadequate, improved provision has been made in maternity and child care facilities to enable mothers to continue to work, but little emphasis has been put upon assisting with the care of elderly relatives for the woman who wishes to continue in a supportive capacity while still fulfilling her own personal and professional potential.

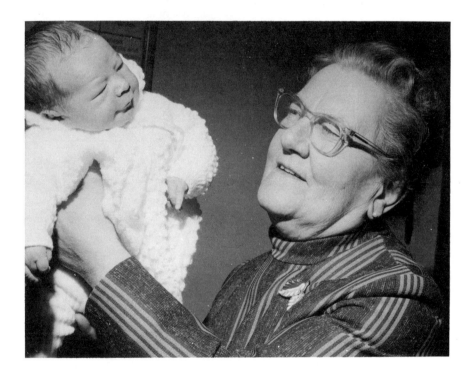

References

1. Laslett, P., The history of ageing and the aged. In Carver, V. and Liddiard, P. (editors), *An Ageing Population*, Open University Press, p.12, 1983
2. Comfort, A., *A Good Age*, Mitchell Beazley, p.171, 1977

Further reading

Garrett, G., Family care and the elderly, *Nursing*, **2**, No. 36, April, 1985, 1061–1063

Means, R. and Smith, R., *The Development of Welfare Services for Elderly People*, Croom Helm, 1985

Townsend, P., *The Family Life of Old People*, Penguin Books, 1963

Finch, J. and Groves, G. (editors), *A Labour of Love: Women, Work and Caring*, Routledge and Kegan Paul, 1983

Chapter 7   Health services approach

The term 'geriatrics' was first coined by Nascher at the turn of the century, deriving from the Greek *geras* — old age — and *iatros* — physician. The work of Dr Marjorie Warren is generally regarded as the basis upon which this 'branch of general medicine concerned with the clinical, social, preventive and remedial aspects of illness in the elderly'[1] has been developed in the UK.

In pre-NHS days the voluntary hospitals dealt primarily with the young and acutely sick, while the elderly, chronically ill patients were relegated to municipal units; it was such a unit, housing 874 old people, that Dr Warren took over in 1935 and transformed in a decade into an active geriatric unit. In 1946 she wrote in the *Lancet*:[2] 'This branch of medicine forms an important subject for the teaching of medical students and should form part of their curriculum; the care of the chronically sick patient should be an essential part of training of student and assistant nurses.' The medical establishment reacted more quickly than the nursing: in 1949 the care of the elderly was included as a university teaching subject and, although perhaps little emphasis was put upon it initially, many dedicated geriatricians have persisted and gained for their speciality not only clinical but also academic respectability and acclaim. There were fourteen professorial units by 1983 dealing with geriatric medicine in the UK.

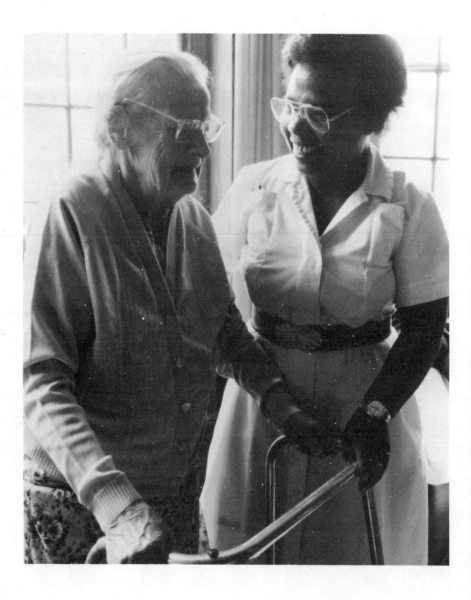

In some areas of the medical world, however, old ideas die hard and high-calibre staff have not always been available in the speciality. At the end of September 1984, 10% of geriatric consultant posts were unfilled, and to meet the Department of Health and Social Security target of one for every 10 000 people over 65 the number of consultant posts would have to be more than doubled.[3] However, a very positive step has been the institution of the Diploma of Geriatric Medicine from the Royal College of Physicians at the end of 1985, intended for hospital doctors in departments of geriatric medicine and general practitioners in training posts.

The feeling that the care of the elderly constituted a professional backwater appeared to persist among nurses for many years, with only a few notable exceptions; the outstanding exception was, and is, Doreen Norton,[4] who, in 1954, was describing the 'challenge to nursing' the elderly presented and who continues to champion their cause today. It is a sad reflection on our profession that it has been outside pressure following national scandals (such as that subsequent to the publication of Barbara Robbs's *Sans Everything*, describing the humiliation and suffering experienced by the elderly in certain 'caring' institutions) rather than heeding the advice of such as Miss Norton that has led to an increased awareness of the nursing needs of older patients and provision for them.

Further to the outcries when such scandalous conditions were revealed, the Hospital Advisory Service was set up in 1969; it was renamed the Health Advisory Service when its remit was broadened in 1976. Independent of the DHSS and reporting directly to the Secretary of State and the Health Authorities concerned, by regular visits of multidisciplinary teams it aims to maintain and improve standards of management and organisation of patient care services mainly for the elderly and the mentally ill. During a visit the existing services are looked at and discussed with clinical staff, and the subsequent written report provides an objective assessment of the services with advice on how staff may constructively build on what they have. The service publishes an annual report with examples of good practice they have found, and can keep government ministers aware of the realities existing in many areas. Most of the visiting team members are clinical workers seconded from NHS positions and can thus have good credence with the staff in the areas concerned.

Dr Warren's advice that geriatric nursing experience should be compulsory for all nurses was echoed by the Royal College of Nursing[5] and the World Health Organization[6] but the statutory body responsible for nurse training was slow to demand allocation for all learners; although pupil nurses have always undertaken such experience, it was not included in the syllabus for students until January 1973 and then it remained optional. Only in July 1979 did it become a definite requirement within the general nursing course (in compliance with the General Nursing Council Educational Policy and the EEC Directives), as did community nursing experience, which encompasses much work with the elderly.

The Joint Board of Clinical Nursing Studies was set up in 1970 and — considered of prime importance by this body — a post-basic course in the nursing care of the elderly was one of the first four courses planned. The first outline curriculum was published in March 1973. The work of the Joint Board was taken over by the National Boards (under the auspices of the United Kingdom Central Council for Nursing and Midwifery) in 1983, and two post-basic courses on the care of the elderly are on offer. Course number 298 is a comprehensive six-month practical and theoretical course for trained nurses; course number 941 is a 22-day course for those with at least two years' experience in the care of the elderly, designed to 'enable registered and enrolled nurses to study new developments based on current research and to update and refresh skills and knowledge in nursing elderly people'. From March 1973 until the end of May 1986, 1048 nurses had undertaken the six-month course and 8020 the shorter one.[7]

In 1976 the Royal College of Nursing set up a Society of Geriatric Nursing, open to all college members, and exceptionally others, working with the elderly in the NHS or in the independent sector. Included in the Society's stated aims are intentions 'to promote awareness within the profession of the expert contribution nurses engaged in this speciality give to the total nursing service' and to promote geriatric nursing to the prominent position it should rightfully occupy. The Society has flourished in the decade since its inception, developing a joint forum with the Society of Psychiatric Nursing, liaising closely with voluntary groups such as Age Concern, and building up a network of 'special interest' groups throughout the country. Regular study days and conferences are arranged, stimulating much interest, and these are of special benefit to nurses working in the smaller independent establishments who may feel isolated from the mainstream of nursing developments in the speciality.

It is interesting that a significant minority of the nurses who choose to work with the elderly are academically as well as practically and professionally able: degree students and graduates frequently recognise the greater opportunities for autonomy, responsibility and initiative involved.[8] It is not a branch of work in which the doctor is necessarily the dominant worker. Several of our leading nurses not only have gained their higher degrees with work on aspects of geriatric nursing, but also have provided us with much valuable research in so doing.

A sizeable body of nursing research with direct bearing on the care of the elderly has now built up, and much has been written in the last few years about services and nursing care, both in specialist journals (such as the *British Journal of Geriatric Nursing*) and in the general nursing press. However, many clinical nurses remain wary of research, with its ivory tower image, and much that has emerged has yet to be acted upon. Ongoing in-service education of nurses in posts in geriatric wards and departments is vital if such problems are to be overcome.

References

1. Pinel, C., Geriatrics as a speciality, *Nursing Times*, **72**, No. 41, 1976, 1601
2. Warren, M., The care of the chronic aged sick, *Lancet*, **i**, 1946, 841
3. *All our Tomorrows: Growing Old in Britain*, Report of the BMA Board of Science and Education, 1986
4. Norton, D., A challenge to nursing, *Nursing Times*, **50**, 1954, 1253
5. Royal College of Nursing Comment on the Report of the Committee on Nursing 1973, Royal College of Nursing and the National Council of Nurses of the United Kingdom, 1973
6. *Planning and Organisation of Geriatric Services*, WHO, 1974
7. Personal communication, ENB Records and Examinations Department
8. Redfern, S., Nursing care of the elderly in hospital, *British Journal of Geriatric Nursing*, **2**, No. 3, 1983, 8–12.

Further reading

British Geriatric Society and Royal College of Nursing, *Improving Care of the Elderly in Hospital,* Royal College of Nursing, London, 1987

Fergus Anderson, W., The evolution of services in the United Kingdom. In Kinnaid, J., Brotheston, J. and Williamson, J. (editors), *The Provision of Care for the Elderly,* Churchill Livingstone, 1985

Part 3 Sharing the Caring

Chapter 8   Community care

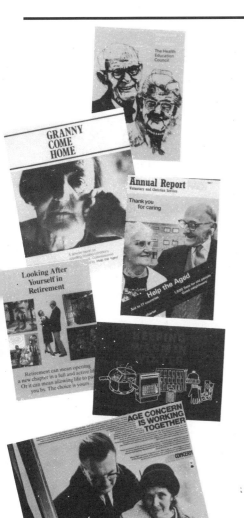

Maintenance of health and independence

An almost universal desire in ageing is the preservation of one's independence and individuality. Society places great emphasis on the development of these qualities in early life and, having attained them and exercised them throughout maturity, one is loath to part with them in old age.

PAUSE FOR THOUGHT

The Shorter Oxford Dictionary defines the two terms as follows:

'Independence' — not depending on another for validity; unwillingness to be under obligation to others.
'Individuality' — separateness of existence, individual character, especially when strongly marked.

Using these definitions, how would you describe your expression of these attributes?

While in any civilised society one must have regard for others, as a healthy mature person one is able to fulfil one's physical and intellectual needs largely distinct from them. The dependence upon others for food and shelter, for example, at its height in infancy and childhood, is minimal in the working adult, whose remuneration enables him to provide his own nutritional and housing requirements; the 'security' of the immediate family is stifling unless extended in the developing years to include free intercourse with others and 'belonging' needs in maturity are satisfied by affiliating oneself with organisations, clubs or societies of one's choice.

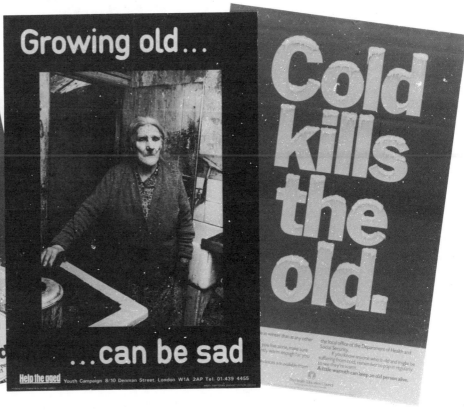

It is this comparative freedom of choice — for most of us there will always be certain restraints in terms of finances or opportunity — that permits us our individuality. Perhaps having experimented with others first, we adopt a certain lifestyle, living where and as we please; we use our leisure time in pursuits which we enjoy. Everything about us, from the face and the dress which we present to the world to the food we select at the supermarket and the manner in which we spend a Sunday morning, indicates something of our individual character.

Why then are the elderly at risk of losing these attributes? Basically there are two possible reasons; firstly, the ageing processes and the illnesses associated with later life may lead to physical frailty and mental decline, rendering the older person less able to cope unaided with the activities of everyday and social living; secondly, his retirement from a conventionally productive and supportive role may, in Western society, relegate him to second-class citizenship in reduced circumstances. Both factors must be actively combated; the maintenance of independence and individuality in the elderly is essential in that dignity and self-respect emanate from their recognition.

While independent living in the community is maintained, individuality is more readily expressed. For such independence, however, there are three basic prerequisites — health adequacy, a suitable environment and a degree of social support — and their provision and promotion are vital considerations.

(a) Health adequacy

Health education generally can be considered from three viewpoints — primary, secondary and tertiary. Primary health education is directed towards the avoidance of disease or injury and the promotion of positive health. Through a variety of techniques the population is encouraged to participate in those activities known to be beneficial to health and to avoid those known to be injurious. Secondary health education is concerned with the early detection of signs of ill-health and its aim is to intervene rapidly where these are found in order to prevent illness or to lessen the possible consequences of it. Tertiary education is that instituted following disease or injury to encourage return to as independent an existence as possible.

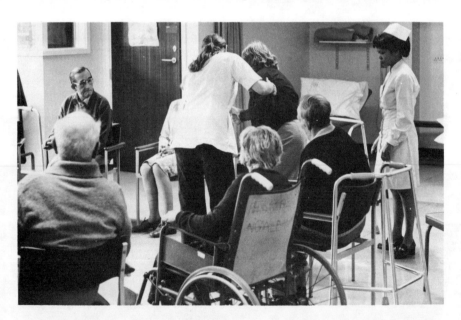

While certain aspects of primary health education are applicable at any age (e.g. the need to reduce an excessive alcohol intake or to give up smoking), for the most part the elderly are the recipients more of secondary or tertiary. Opportunities for such education are many — in Pre-Retirement Courses, through the mass media, in social clubs and day centres and on a one-to-one basis whenever the older person has any contact with any member of the Primary Health Care Team (see following section (b)). In an article on health promotion in the elderly, Patricia Best[1] has pointed out that this age group is often more amenable to such teaching than the younger generation — their survival in so rapidly changing a society has depended upon adaptability, which she sees as frequently demonstrated in this respect.

Professor Brocklehurst[2] has suggested that in terms of health education for the elderly there are three special areas of concern — retirement and its implications, the high incidence of unreported ill-health and the problems consequent upon ageing and the environment. Retirement and primary education to prevent associated problems has been discussed in an earlier chapter; let us now consider health screening as an aspect of secondary education and environmental adaptation as an aspect of tertiary education.

Many older people, and also their relatives, have a low expectation of health in old age and frequently untoward symptoms are put down to the age factor alone. Over the last decade or so several studies in different communities have found much ill-health, unknown to the person's general practitioner, seriously impairing the quality of life — problems such as depression, foot problems leading to immobility, visual and hearing impairment restricting social activity; problems which would have been amenable to treatment.

Further to these studies, many health care teams have instituted a screening system for the elderly, and some also for the middle-aged, in an attempt to encourage them to reach old age rather more healthily. Age/sex registers are obtained by the general practitioner from the family practitioner committee and appointments are offered to all the people on the list within the appropriate age group; failure to accept the invitiation can be followed up by the community nurse or health visitor to ensure that its purpose was understood and to discuss it further if desired.

The initial assessment offered is very comprehensive, covering social as well as physical health, and the former — in terms of nutrition, smoking, functional ability within the home, etc. — is generally assessed by the nurse members of the team in the home before the person is seen by the doctor. Observations of temperature, pulse rate and blood pressure are recorded, a sample of urine is obtained for routine analysis and blood for estimation of haemoglobin is taken; height and weight are noted and an electrocardiogram recorded. A simple self-assessment questionnaire is often used to indicate any particular anxieties which the person would like to discuss on his examination.

Following screening any problems encountered can be acted upon as appropriate: chiropody can be arranged, for example, or advice can be given on weight reduction; anaemia can be investigated and therapy instituted as required. Plans can then be made for further checks; where no immediate problems are apparent and none foreseen in the reasonable future, follow-up may be annually by the nursing staff with referral to the doctor as necessary.

Where the ageing processes or age-related disorders have taken their toll on an elderly person, education in the adaptation of the home environment to counteract disability assumes importance. The control of posture deteriorates with ageing and there is an increased likelihood of falls with subsequent injury; the likelihood is compounded by badly lit stairways, loose rugs or carpets, poorly sited plugs and such. As the body's heat-regulating centre becomes less efficient problems may again arise unless suitable modification of the environment is undertaken, in this instance because of hypothermia, or occasionally hyperthermia. If bladder function is impaired judicious siting of a commode or reorganisation of living accommodation to enable easier access to toilet facilities is essential if incontinence is not to ensue. The opportunities in this area for health promotion are legion.

(b) A suitable environment

In the foregoing paragraph the elderly person's environment was considered in terms of adaptation to accommodate disability; it is necessary also to consider it in its wider, extended sense when thinking broadly of maintaining independence. The majority of older people depend upon public transport, and facilities such as shops, post offices, doctors' surgeries and chemists must be realistically sited if they are to manage unaided. All too often these factors would appear not to have been taken into account in new developments; the same difficulties may be experienced in older residential areas as well, however, with the building of new health centres necessitating the closure of branch surgeries and corner shops giving way to large central supermarkets.

Increasingly over recent years older owner-occupiers have experienced difficulties maintaining their homes in later life. About half of the elderly own their own homes and the problems associated with repairs, decoration and general upkeep may assume unmanageable proportions. Some of these difficulties are outlined in Muir Gray's excellent article[3] 'Problems for the property owning democracy'.

Until now there has been no research into the direct effects of housing on the health of elderly people which groups could usefully employ in attempting to obtain better conditions in either the public or the private sector.[4] With the assistance of general practitioners, the Institute of Environmental Health conducted a nationwide survey (Summer 1986) and the results are awaited with interest. However, most community workers appreciate that many elderly people may be seriously handicapped by their home environment, because of the factors indicated in Table 8.1.[5]

Table 8.1 The national picture of housing and the elderly

- A quarter of all households are now 'elderly only'.
- Nearly three million elderly people live alone and just over a third are 75 or over.
- The number of people aged 75 or over is predicted to rise to over 4 million by 2011.
- Half of elderly people already own their own homes and are therefore responsible for any repairs or improvements that are necessary.
- 389 000 people of pensionable age (1981 census) have no toilet inside their homes; just under half of them are in owner-occupied housing.
- 283 000 (or 27%) of properties needing over £7000 of repairs are occupied by elderly households (1981 House Condition Survey).
- 473 000 (or 43%) of all unfit properties are occupied by elderly households (1981 survey).

While a move to sheltered accommodation (see later in this chapter) may be the solution for some elderly people, advice on and help with improving their homes may be more appropriate for others. Obviously, with a low income and dwindling savings this may be difficult, but recent research has shown that with professional support it is certainly feasible. Outlined in Table 8.2 are some of the sources of help that may be available.[5]

Table 8.2 What help is available?

- Housing advice from the local authority (for example, a housing aid centre), a local housing association, Citizens Advice Bureau (CAB) or local branch of Age Concern.
- Community occupational therapists in the social services department can give advice on aids and adaptations.
- Improvement grant officer in the housing or environmental health department can give advice on grant aid for repairs, improvements or adaptations.
- Local building society branch managers should be able to advise on improvement mortgages. These are available on an interest-only basis and are known as interest-only mortgages or maturity loans. These mortgages are available for owner-occupiers over 60 with capital repayment deferred until the house is sold or inherited. Mortgages can be used on their own or to top up a grant.
- Welfare rights office (or the local DHSS) can give advice on single payments (lump sums) available in some cases, for small repairs, and help with the interest charge on the improvement mortgage for some elderly people in receipt of (or eligible for) supplementary benefit.*
- Agency services for elderly owner-occupiers — known as Staying Put or Care and Repair schemes — are provided in some areas of the country.
- CABs or local authority housing departments should know what is available in individual areas.

  * Supplementary benefit and home improvement grants are under review by central government and there are likely to be radical changes.

Professionals must beware when considering the suitability of an old person's environment that they do not make value judgements based on their own standards, especially in relation to cleanliness and safety. In the final analysis the criteria for judging the adequacy of the home must be those of the old person himself; familiarity and valued associations may make up tenfold for the inconvenience of an outside toilet or a damp bathroom. Some degree of risk is inevitable in all our lives and the degree of risk to which an informed elderly person knowingly subjects himself must be his decision.

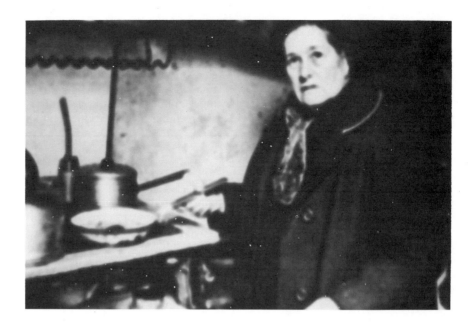

(c) Social support

Living alone may prove no problem to the younger elderly person, especially if this has been the style of most of his adult life; the older elderly person, however, deprived of his spouse or a nearby family, is particularly vulnerable where social support is not available to encourage independence. The support systems are outlined in the next section; they include provisions within the home of a domestic and personal nature, and outside it in relation to involvement in social and community activities. They have many advantages for the client group they serve, and have been found to be viable alternatives to rehousing, with all its attendant problems. However, they are not cheap to set up or to run, but they are certainly less expensive than rehousing and are generally much preferred by the elderly people themselves.

References

1. Best, P., Health promotion in the elderly, in *The Elderly: A Challenge to Nursing*, Nursing Times Publication, 1978
2. Brocklehurst, J.C., Health education in the elderly, *Journal of the Institute of Health Education*, **14,** Part 4, 1976, 115–120
3. Muir Gray, J.A., Problems for the property owning democracy, *New Age*, Winter 1980/81, 24–27
4. Editorial in *Community Outlook*. With *Nursing Times*, February, 1986
5. Wheeler, R., Staying put, *Community Outlook*. With *Nursing Times*, February, 1986

Further reading

Wheeler, R., *Don't Move — We've Got You Covered*, Institute of Housing, London, 1985
Tinker, A., *Staying at Home — Helping Elderly People*, HMSO, 1984
Muir Gray, J.A., Biological ageing and screening. *Nursing*, 2, No. 41, September, 1985, 1227–1229

Provision of community services

No one elderly person is 'typical' or could be said to exhibit 'typical' needs; Mrs Brown, however, has multiple needs occasioned by multiple problems — medical, functional and social — and thus hers is a useful case to consider when thinking of the comprehensive services available to support the elderly in the community.

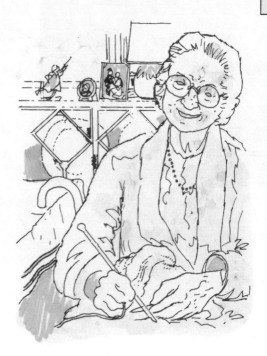

'I was widowed 14 years last December — yes, I was 63 when Jack went; so sudden it was, picture of health one day, gone the next. Of course Stella, my girl, only lived around the corner with the little ones then — they were a great comfort to me, they were. But her husband got moved to Scotland with his job so I see so little of them now — great-grandchildren I've got up there too. She wanted me to go with them when they went but I've been in this house since the day I was wed — we bought it over all those years — and nothing will move me from it. I can get in the garden on a nice day — it was his pride and joy — you should have seen it then, all lawn and roses. There's pictures upstairs of it as it was — I'd show you but I can't get up there now of course. I use the frame all the time now but my bed is down here and I manage.

'I'll make a cup of tea in a minute. What? Oh, my health. Well, I've hd the sugar diabetes for 20 years now — I have the injection every day. They say that's why my sight has gone so bad now — the diabetes. I don't know if it affects the heart too — I have tablets for the failure. And I do feel the cold — but the electric is so dear and I have to be careful with the pension. The Centre is warm when I go there — oh yes, I go twice — Tuesdays — no, Wednesdays and Fridays. The van is chilly on the way but I like to get out to talk to the others — all my neighbours are good but really it's only the cats I've got for proper company.

It's outside if you want to go, dear — you mind the back step. I'll put the kettle on. My Stella always says I make a good cup of tea — that's my girl you know, she lives in Scotland. She used to live round Brandwen Drive when Jack was alive — adored the kids he did. I don't see them much now — I said to the Vicar yesterday, I wish Scotland was in Bath. But I don't complain. They wanted to put me in a home a while back but I told them — this is my home and I'll only go when I go, if you see what I mean. I've had a good life and folk are very kind.'

For ease of description here Mrs Brown's needs are divided into physical, functional and social (Table 8.3); the distinction between them is somewhat arbitrary, however, since health is dependent upon social welfare and vice versa in the community situation.

Table 8.3   The needs of Mrs Brown

Physical	Functional	Social
Medical treatment of physical disease Supervision of medical treatment (drug therapy, urine testing, insulin administration, dietary provision) Assistance with personal needs (hygiene, foot care)	Provision of 'extended' personal care — collection of pension and shopping, nutritional needs, housework and laundry, gardening and decorating	Financial assistance Opportunities for social stimulation and involvement

The support network which keeps Mrs Brown in the community by fulfilling these needs is extensive and the roles of the 'carers' sometimes overlap, depending on the availability or otherwise of personnel, as will be seen in the description that follows. The account also gives the lie to the myth that community care is less expensive than hospital or residential care; where this is so it is generally because the client is receiving inadequate support.

(a) Mrs Brown's support network

Once a month Mrs Brown is visited by her GP and every two months she is seen by the Liaison Health Visitor attached to the Diabetic Clinic at the local hospital; she has never really 'come to terms' with her diabetes and was very ready to abandon her daily care to the Community Nurse when her sight began to deteriorate. Every morning her urine is tested by the nurse and her insulin given; on the days when her home care assistant does not visit, the nurse also supervises her breakfast. Although able to wash and dress herself, Mrs Brown is not able to bath unaided and the community auxiliary visits her weekly to assist. As a diabetic she has priority with the chiropodist, who attends to her feet every six weeks on her visit to the day centre.

Mrs Brown's 'extended' personal needs are met by a combination of social services and voluntary provision; as she has lived for nearly sixty years in the same house in an older residential area she is well known and well supported by her neighbours and the local church. She is visited on three days a week by her home care assistant, who shops and cleans for her and attends to the laundry; she supervises her breakfast and prepares an evening meal to leave for her. On those days Mrs Brown has meals-on-wheels at lunch times. On the other two weekdays she has her lunch at the day centre; she has good neighbours living on either side and they take it in turns to prepare an evening meal when she returns from the centre and they also give her her meals at the weekend. Teenagers from the local youth club have recently been visiting twice a month to keep her garden tidy.

The social services support which Mrs Brown receives was organised by the local authority social worker some time ago but she again became involved in her care recently, alerted by the Community Nurse to her client's concern about finances. A rates rebate was applied for and obtained and an application lodged with a trades' society to which Mr Brown had belonged for financial aid for heating improvements; the outcome of this is still awaited.

Either the Vicar or the Deaconess visits Mrs Brown weekly during the winter months but in the better weather transport is arranged to take her to church on Sundays.

The provision of community services will now be considered in rather more general detail and the roles of the personnel involved will be more closely examined.

(b) Health care provision

This can be summarised as shown in Figure 8.1:

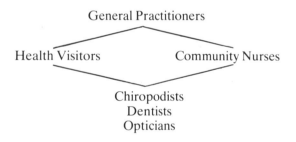

General Practitioners

Health Visitors   Community Nurses

Chiropodists
Dentists
Opticians

Figure 8.1   Summary of health care provision

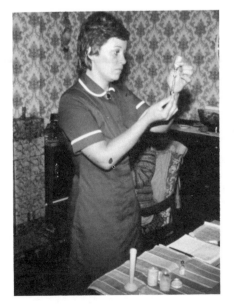

The basic concept underlying the formation in recent years of Primary Health Care Teams is that the varied needs of patients require the concerted skills of a variety of practitioners to meet them. Where the health professionals making up this team — the GP, community nurses and midwives and health visitors — share the same premises some of the physical barriers to communication are obviously lessened, but good working relationships, essential for the ultimate good of the patient, have to be worked on; they depend on each team member appreciating the skills of the others, fully understanding their roles and the need for mutual support.

The GP is responsible for the medical supervision of the patients on his list — an average of between 2000 and 3000 people. A good proportion of his time will be taken up by the elderly patients on this list, especially the older elderly with their relatively higher incidence of need. In recognition of this the general practitioner is paid an additional per capita amount annually for each person over 65 for whom he cares.

Community Nurses — Registered and Enrolled — are responsible for the nursing care of patients on the GPs' lists and some recent estimates have indicated that more than 75% of their time is spent with the elderly.

Leading the nursing team, the District Nursing Sister is responsible for the delivery of skilled care to elderly patients living in the community — in the home, in the health centre and in residential accommodation. She is accountable for the work she delegates in addition to her own.

The functions of the District Nurse have been defined as:[1]

1. Identification of physical, social and emotional needs of patients in their own homes.
2. Planning and provision of appropriate programmes of nursing care, especially for the following groups: the chronically sick, the disabled, the frail elderly, the terminally ill and post-operative patients.
3. Mobilising community resources both professional and voluntary.
4. Identification of the special needs of the carer and the family.
5. Ensuring continuity of care between home and hospital in both directions.
6. Promotion of health education and self-care with individuals and groups.
7. Rehabilitation.
8. Counselling.

Many of the basic personal care components — assisting with getting up, washing and dressing, bathing — are now taken care of by auxiliary staff under the supervision of the trained nurse, freeing the latter to undertake the more skilled aspects of care, to teach family or other carers about general patient management, to counsel and support. The service provides 24-hour cover seven days a week; in some areas a night sitting service is provided for the critically and terminally ill in addition to the trained staff on call for emergencies.

Over the last decade District Nurses have been having to provide more care for more patients because of changes in the number of hospital beds available, the policy of earlier discharge and the increased use of residential accommodation, in addition to changing population characteristics. In some areas this has led to a serious mismatch between the increase in the patients needing nursing care and the supply of District Nurses available, with very large case loads and many attendant problems resulting.

The aim of the Health Visitor in relation to the care of the elderly is to maintain healthy, independent living in the home situation for as long as is possible. Trained in preventive health care, she is responsible for health promotion through group and individual teaching and counselling, surveillance of those in need and liaison with other agencies or organisations as appropriate; her involvement in screening programmes was discussed in the previous section.

Some Health Visitors act in a liaison capacity between hospital geriatric departments and the community and this service has greatly benefited many patients in ensuring a smooth transition from in-patient to home care. Few areas, however, are yet able to meet the guidelines of one Health Visitor to 3000 population; in an effort to make certain that those really in need of support receive it, some districts maintain an 'Elderly at Risk' register, with those on it being visited regularly; 'risk factors' include living alone after the age of 75, having a chronic illness or disability, having recently been bereaved or living in substandard housing accommodation.

However, because of their statutory responsibility for mothers and children under 5, not infrequently the care of the elderly assumes low priority in the Health Visitors' eyes, and in many cases much of their work with them has been found to be delegated to Health Assistants, usually registered nurses with no Health Visitor training.[2] Sadly, this would appear to be supported by the Health Visitors' Association, whose document *Health Visiting in the Eighties* sees only a limited role for its members with the elderly and makes no mention of their specific educational and preventive skills with them. Some specialist workers, such as Liz Day, have challenged[3] such assumptions and have made important contributions, but with changing demographic and health care trends attitudinal alteration in the profession as a whole with a consequent change in practice is seen by many to be essential. Others argue that all work with the elderly — preventive as well as therapeutic — should be the province of the District Nurse, with Health

Visitors left concentrating their attention on child care. Sadly, while the debate continues in the profession, unmet needs continue to exist among the elderly in question.

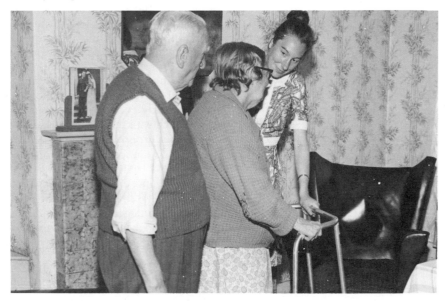

Some Primary Health Care Teams have a direct social work attachment and the social worker may actually share the Health Centre premises. Again this militates in favour of much improved communication but as yet it is not a common feature.

Other health professionals working in the community with special relevance to the elderly are chiropodists, dentists and opticians. Chiropody services are free under the NHS and ideally the elderly in need of foot care should receive it every six to eight weeks; in practice, however, it is in very short supply and certain groups, such as patients with diabetes, have priority. Where simple pedicure only is required for a patient unable to manage unaided, the Community Nurse will undertake the task; for more complex treatments appointments will be made at Health Centres or Day Centres or occasionally a domiciliary visit may be arranged. Many elderly people resort to private chiropody where waiting lists are prohibitively long.

Patients do not register with a dentist in the same way that they do with a general practitioner; each course of treatment comes under a new 'contract' between the two. Increasingly, elderly patients are facing considerable difficulty, as many dentists are no longer prepared to accept NHS patients, only those who are willing and able to pay for private treatment. Where he is fortunate enough to be seen as an NHS patient, the elderly person is eligible for two free examinations annually and, if he is in receipt of supplementary pension, to any necessary treatment to either natural teeth or dentures.

Annual eye examinations by opticians are free, as are any others clinically necessary between yearly visits. Again, if the elderly patient receives supplementary pension, he is entitled to free spectacles or other low-vision aids; a standard charge is otherwise made under NHS provision or frames and/or lenses may be purchased privately.

(c) Social services provision

The personal social services are under the control of the local authorities and have four main areas of responsibility:

1. Services in the home.
2. Services in the community.
3. Provision of residential accommodation.
4. Provision of information on other services.

Social workers are employed by the Social Work Department and may work either directly from it or by attachment to Primary Health Care Teams. They are responsible for assessing clients' needs in the community and organising intervention as indicated in relation to the services mentioned above; studies have indicated that, from the elderly consumers' point of view, this is where their value lies — in the provision of positive practical help rather than in the somewhat nebulous generalised visiting at which volunteers are likely to be more acceptable and successful.

Perhaps the two best-known services available to elderly clients in their own homes are the home care assistants (formerly home helps) and meals-on-wheels. The compass of the home care assistant's work is wide; her most common task is cleaning but frequently she also does the washing and ironing, shopping and some cooking or preparing of meals. Each client's ability to pay for the service is assessed by the local organiser but many home care assistants visit for more hours than they are paid for, returning to ensure that all is well in the evening or over the weekend. They are often the people with whom elderly clients living alone have most contact and as such they may get in touch with the social worker or community nurse should the need arise.

Another group of carers currently being introduced experimentally in some areas, and mentioned here to distinguish them from home care assistants, are home aides. Their allocation to a newly discharged client is of shorter duration (usually no more than six weeks) but on a more intensive and personal level; the intention is that, by providing support for perhaps six to eight hours daily at first, independence can be regained as it is gradually withdrawn. Home aides generally have their base in social services departments and they are local authority funded.

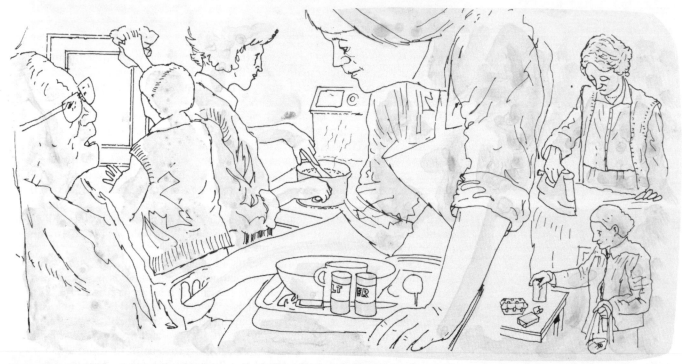

To return to social services provision — the second most common service is 'meals-on-wheels'. The idea originated by the Women's Voluntary Service (now the Women's Royal Voluntary Service) during the last war has now largely been taken over by the local authorities, who deliver to the client's home a hot, two-course meal on a certain number of days weekly. Some luncheon clubs for the elderly are also supplied with meals from the same service; since meals in most societies fulfil social as well as physical needs, the stimulation of others' company and group involvement is beneficial especially for those living alone. Transport is frequently a problem, however, unless volunteer drivers can be recruited for this purpose, as many clients are unable to make their own way to the clubs.

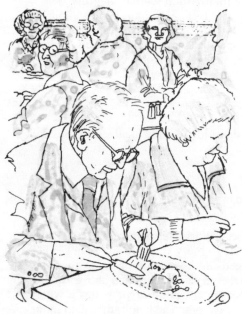

Domiciliary occupational therapists are based in social services departments and can be contacted to assess the capabilities of the elderly person in relation to the activities of everyday living in the home. Under the 1970 Chronically Sick and Disabled Persons Act local authorities are then able to make alterations to the home on the therapist's recommendation and any aids to enable easier living can be installed — these may include supportive rails by toilet or bath or kitchen aids for the elderly disabled housewife; they are tailored to meet individual needs. Telephones can be requested and installed free of charge for the elderly client who lives alone and who may, for medical reasons, need to summon help; these are currently in short supply, however.

Perhaps the most important community facility for which the social services departments have responsibility is day centre provision. Designed as social centres, some are also associated with the 'Employment Fellowship', which, through negotiation with local manufacturers, provides regular basic work with some small financial remuneration. In diversional therapy others may make their own products for local sale. Day centre provision has been badly affected by the current financial stringencies, however, and transport difficulties are again an ever-present problem.

The third area of social services responsibility — the provision of residential accommodation — will be considered in the next section. The fourth is making known to elderly clients information on other services available in the community and the entitlements to which they may be due — perhaps rent or rates rebates or additional DHSS pensions or allowances. The manner in which the information is given is of paramount importance; many of the elderly — and especially the very elderly — are reluctant to claim what is seen as 'charity', but what is in reality a benefit for which they have contributed over a lifetime.

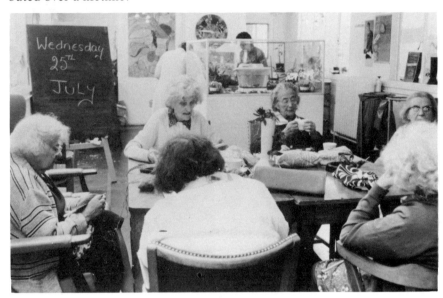

(d) Voluntary provision

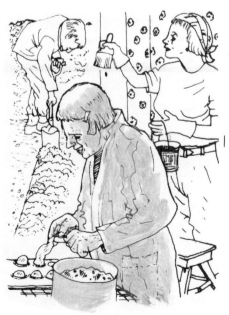

Perhaps the most important and effective group of community carers has been left until last — the vast army of friends, neighbours and voluntary workers without whom the services for the elderly in the UK would be not only impoverished but also immobilised. In some instances the 'good neighbour' relationship has been formalised, the local authority paying a small weekly amount to those willing to help out an elderly person, but in the great majority of cases the shopping, gardening, giving of lifts and general support is a spontaneous response to need.

Much emphasis in the past has been on the voluntary support given by school and college students, but, as Robin Webster (the Director of Age Concern, Scotland) has pointed out,[4] the requisite 'wisdom, initiative, commitment and enthusiasm are certainly not the prerogative of the young' and the younger, often newly retired elderly can make a significant contribution. Often the friendship of someone more of their own age and background may be more acceptable to the older person and, with the young being a more rapidly shifting population, such a relationship is likely to be more enduring.

Whatever their origin, however, WRVS, Red Cross, Task Force or Church organisation, volunteers have been seen[5] to be used to maximum advantage in the following areas:

1. Supporting the care normally given by relatives, friends or neighbours — especially when the latter are on holiday or away for other reasons.
2. Visiting the lonely and house-bound with a view, if possible, to integrating them into appropriate clubs or day centres. Acting as links between statutory organisations and community groups.
3. Within residential or day care settings acting as 'animateurs', helping the elderly maintain their independence by keeping up their activities or interests of younger days.

Lastly, mention must be made of the self-help groups organised by the elderly for their mutual benefit. The best-known of these is probably the 'Link Scheme' begun in 1975 with the support of Age Concern and the Pre-Retirement Association but now largely locally organised around the country. Services are rendered in return for other services rendered, with stamp tokens used to indicate the number of hours' work involved; for example, an elderly woman may bake in return for assistance with gardening, or household repairs may be undertaken in exchange for sewing or washing. Such domestic skills are the ones most commonly available but more varied ones — language teaching, roofing, car maintenance — may also be on offer. In some areas all age groups are involved in the scheme, with younger members able to offer assistance with more strenuous tasks such as decorating in return for babysitting or knitting. Of the many benefits of the scheme, perhaps the most important is the recognition of one's own skills as valued in an exchange relationship.

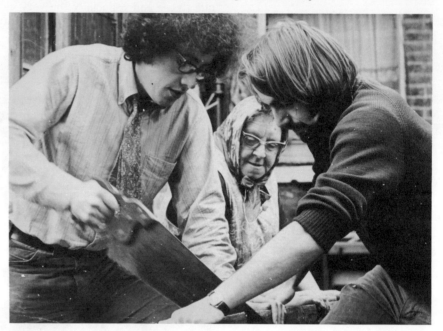

References

1. Ross, F.M., Nursing old people in the community. In Redfern, S. (editor), *Nursing Elderly People*, Churchill Livingstone, p. 342, 1986
2. Dunnell, K. and Dobbs, J., *Nurses Working in the Community*, Office of Population Censuses and Surveys, HMSO, 1982
3. Day, L., Health visiting the elderly in the 80's — do we care enough? *Health Visitor*, **54**, No. 12, 1981, 538–539
4. 'The new man in Scotland' — Interview with Robin Webster, *New Age*, Winter, 1980, 32
5. Cypher, J., Support and care, *New Age*, Spring, 1981, 22–23

Further reading

While, A.E., Health visiting and the elderly. In Redfern, S. (editor), *Nursing Elderly People*, Churchill Livingstone, Chapter 27, 1986

Phillipson, C., Health visiting and older people: a review of current trends, *Health Visitor*, **58**, No. 12, 1985, 357–358.

Ross, F.M., Nursing old people in the community. In Redfern, S. (editor), *Nursing Elderly People,* Churchill Livingstone, Chapter 26, 1986

Garrett, G., Pensions and benefits for the elderly and their carers, *Professional Nurse*, November, 1985, 45–46

When the time comes . . .

Very many elderly will live out their days happily independent, still contributing more to the community than they have ever taken from it; others will maintain a 'supported independence' in their own homes with family and friends, voluntary and statutory agencies providing social or practical help as is individually indicated. For a proportion of the elderly, however, residual problems following illness or the frailty of advancing years will mean that coping alone is no longer feasible and the time will come when alternatives must be sought.

(a) Living with relatives

Who are the relatives with whom the more dependent elderly live? It is a common supposition that they are primarily the offspring of the older person but this is very often not the case; a recent survey in an urban area[1] showed that 30% of those over 75 had had no children and 45% had had only one or two — since some of the latter had outlived these offspring, a total of 35% therefore had no living child at all. This figure has been reflected in other surveys around Great Britain.

Where couples grow old together one partner in later life frequently has charge of the other in illness or infirmity; it is most often the wife (generally younger and fitter) who must assume the role of carer but many elderly men also devotedly tend those they took 'for better, for worse . . . in sickness and in health'. In the absence of a spouse, a brother or sister may act in a supporting capacity or a close friend of the same age.

When an elderly person does have children, by the time he has reached advanced old age, the children themselves may be past retirement and their own health and resources less than satisfactory. Where adult children are younger, although their health and coping ability may be assumed to be less taxed, their parents' time of need frequently coincides with the time when they are most deeply committed elsewhere — to their own offspring, career or community — and there may well be a resulting conflict, in some instances almost impossible to resolve and adversely affecting family relationships for years to come.

1 Situations occasioning the move

Where an agreement has been reached in healthier days that a joint home would be acceptable to both parties, fewer problems are likely to arise and indeed mutual benefits may come out of the situation. Help with gardening or decorating, babysitting and childminding services may be seen as a fair exchange for cooking and laundry and — especially where a degree of privacy and independence can be ensured by the provision of a 'granny flat' or annexe — family relationships may be strengthened by the move.

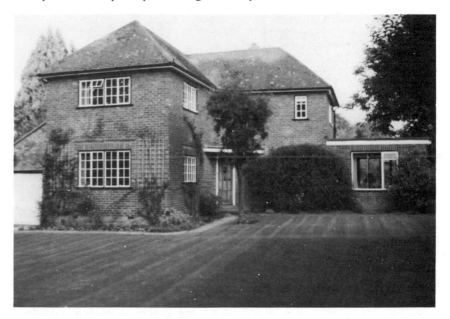

In the case of the more disabled elderly, however, two situations commonly occasion such a move. Months of slow decline during which all the supportive services have been involved may culminate in a situation which cannot be allowed to continue as it is in no way satisfactory or safe for the elderly person. Alternatively, an emergency situation may arise with the rapid deterioration of the older person's health or the illness or death of the usual carer. Since decisions made hastily may be ill-informed and emotionally swayed, in the latter instance temporary 'holding' measures are better employed than irrevocably permanent ones such as selling up a home and all that this entails.

Before long-term decisions are made, open and honest discussion should take place concerning the needs and prospective problems of both the elderly person and the potential carer and any other concerned parties; the general practitioner, health visitor or social worker should preferably be present at such a discussion or their advice and guidance should be sought beforehand. However, any tendency to make arrangements for, rather than with, the elderly person in respect of her future should be strongly resisted unless mental functioning is seriously impaired. Neither age nor physical frailty renders a person incapable of rational insight into situations and justifiable resentment on the elderly person's part may wreck plans formulated without her knowledge or agreement.

Whenever a decision is reached and arrangements are made to take an elderly person into the family home or when an adult child returns to the parental home in a caring capacity, all appropriate supportive services (such as meals-on-wheels, day centre provision, holiday relief) should be mobilised from the start so that the situation is seen to be manageable and anxiety, depression and guilt do not rapidly ensue in the carer or, indeed, in the elderly person herself.

PAUSE FOR THOUGHT

Below are the outlines of two situations in which daughters assumed responsibility for the care of disabled elderly parents.

What potential difficulties can you identify for the elderly people themselves and for their carers in these situations?

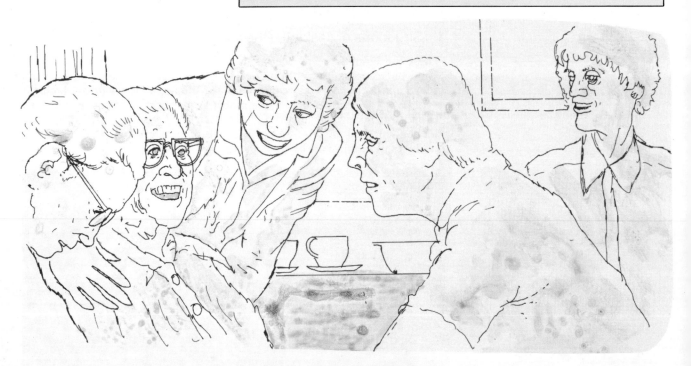

(a) Jean Greenwood, a 47-year-old part-time teacher, was married to a lecturer in the field of further education; their two sons aged 16 and 17 were still at school when Jean's 77-year-old widowed mother, who suffered from angina, had a total hip replacement and was no longer able to manage in her flat. She decided to offer her mother a home with her family in their three-bedroomed bungalow a short distance away and to give up teaching in order to care for her.

(b) Lorraine Henderson had been the only child of older parents. At 30, she was a personnel officer with a publishing company, she owned her own flat and led an active social life during the week; at weekends she returned to her parent's home some 60 miles away to help her mother

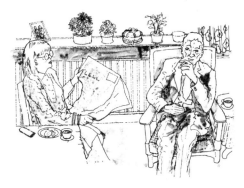

care for her father, who had had several strokes. When her mother, quite unexpectedly, collapsed and died, she discussed with her father either returning to the parental home or making a new home for them both near to her place of work. After some thought, he agreed to move; her flat and his house were sold and a bungalow bought into which they settled.

Three-generational life is rarely completely harmonious and many factors in the first instance militate against it being so here. In a three-bedroom house, the most likely solution to the space problem would involve Jean's two sons sharing a room at a stage when privacy and 'personal space' are vital to adolescents. No doubt their way of life could also cause their grandmother some distress, with loud music, numerous friends on motorbikes and late nights all being possible causes of friction.

For Jean herself, giving up paid employment would mean loss of income, independence and social contacts; menopausal problems may be exacerbated by these factors in addition to the increased workload involved in caring for her mother. Weekends away and holidays may be curtailed unless alternative arrangements can be made for her mother and any marital friction may be highlighted by the conflicting demands of the new situation.

Belonging to a generation in which few married women worked outside the home and in which ideas on child rearing were totally different from today's, Jean's mother might well not appreciate the frustrations she may experience in her changed circumstances and she may be confused or alarmed by the apparently *laissez-faire* attitude taken towards the grandchildren's behaviour. Unless a definite and purposeful role — taking into account her physical limitations — can be worked out for her, she may feel totally extraneous to the life of the household. Obviously a degree of tolerance and adaptation on her part will be called for but she should be encouraged to preserve those aspects of her old lifestyle and outlook important to her. Thus the same degree of adaptation and tolerance will be demanded of the younger generations.

In the second instance, the most immediate and important problem for both Lorraine and her father would be their bereavement experience; for her father, the loss of a much loved wife at the time of his own failing health and considerable disability may render him unwilling or unable to look constructively to the future. For Lorraine, the practical problems involved in arranging the sales of the house and flat, of organising a new home and shouldering the total responsibility for her father's care may of necessity take precedence over working through such an emotional trauma, with her unresolved grief then a problem in the months or years to come.

Wherever possible, single sons or daughters caring for elderly parents should continue to work as they are able, for both financial and personal reasons. The difficulties inherent in doing so are obvious, however, and Lorraine, as well as having the additional workload when at home, would have the anxiety when at work as to her father coping alone. Full-time employment combined with long-term caring is extremely tiring and the opportunities for social relaxation are greatly curtailed — entertaining friends at home may be difficult and going out more so.

Professional development may not be easy for Lorraine, with further courses posing problems and moves to other areas being out of the question; any close relationships may be hampered by both practical and emotional considerations.

For her father the prospect of approaching a new life 60 miles from old friends and acquaintances when his mobility is limited may be daunting in the extreme. An over-dependence on Lorraine's help and support with unreasonable demands on her time and affection may ensue; alternatively he may vent his anger and frustration upon her and attempt to reassert the parental dominance of earlier years.

These then are the potential difficulties that may arise in the given circumstances. However, the positive possibilities should also be envisaged if a one-sided picture is not to be given. Family relationships rarely change dramatically in later years and where individuals have got on well beforehand, sensitive to and adapting to each other's needs and lifestyle, the pattern is often maintained. In the second instance, for example, once the inevitable teething problems of adjusting to the new situation are overcome, if the relationship in earlier years has been open and mutually supportive, Lorraine's father may well develop as encouraging and understanding an attitude to her needs as she to his.

While no family environment can be totally problem-free (nor would this be desirable — the human spirit demands a certain degree of mental and emotional tussle!), what are the important considerations in achieving as mutually satisfying a situation as possible where a disabled elderly person is cared for by relatives? Perhaps these should be looked at under psychological, practical and financial headings.

Independence and individuality have been considered previously (p. 37); when the older person's ability to cope independently is reduced and he is cared for by another, unless strenuous efforts are made on both sides to preserve individuality, interdependence may result with a blurring or diminution of the personalities to the detriment of both — especially to the carer, who must resume her own life on the demise of the elder. However severe the older person's disability, independent functioning should be encouraged to the maximum and as much of the usual lifestyle as is feasible should be maintained by both parties; support by other relatives and outside agencies in the form of transport or visiting or sitting-in will make this more realistic in order that an acceptable quality of life may be enjoyed.

However good the relationship there will almost invariably come a time in a prolonged caring situation when both parties need a time away from each other and the home environment. Where other relatives are not available or not able to assist, 'holiday relief' may be afforded by the elderly person 'boarding out' with other families (in schemes such as that run by the Liverpool Personal Service Society) or by short-term admission to residential care facilities. In many areas the Red Cross runs holiday schemes for the disabled elderly in seaside or country areas.

Practical considerations in a caring situation include the provision of a suitable environment which encourages independence and reduces the demands of the carer; these points are of special importance when immobility or incontinence are problems. In the former case, assessment by the domiciliary occupational therapist and the provision of aids as appropriate are vital, with the carer and the elderly person being instructed in their use; in the latter, the provision of an incontinence service (covering the distribution and disposal of pads, other appliances and bed linen) may mean the difference between the family coping effectively and their requesting admission to hospital. Sadly, at the time of writing, this type of service is not widely available.

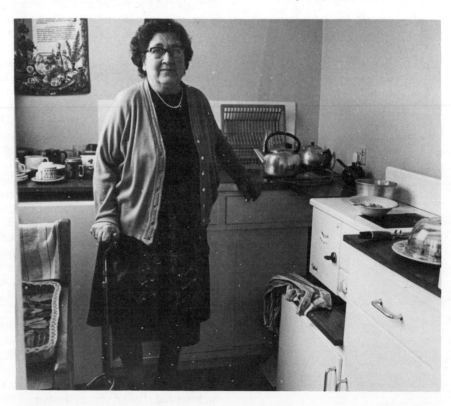

Financially a family may be disadvantaged when supporting an elderly relative at home. There may be loss of income when the principal carer is required to give up paid employment, or additional heating and food costs combined with the need to acquire such labour-saving devices as washing machines or tumble driers may pose problems. It is essential therefore that the elderly and their families be fully aware of the benefits to which they are entitled; in addition to his retirement pension, the elderly person may be eligible for additional allowances for extra heating, special diet or laundry services. Where he requires attendance at frequent intervals by day or night to ensure his welfare and safety, he is entitled to the Constant Attendance Allowance, which is tax free and non-means tested. The person providing the care for the elderly person claiming this allowance, if of working age but unable to work because of her caring commitment, may be eligible to receive the Invalid Care Allowance.

2 Crisis points

Many families and single carers cope admirably with elderly dependants until a crisis is precipitated by the onset of confusion or incontinence. Since both are symptoms of underlying problems and not diagnoses in themselves and since both may be rapidly remediable with the institution of appropriate therapy (*see* later chapters), the elderly person requires immediate medical investigation, treatment and nursing care until the acute episode is resolved. This may necessitate the temporary admission of the person to hospital but a realistically optimistic view of the situation should be taken with the relatives in order that they may expect and be prepared to receive him home again on his recovery. Obviously a thorough review of the situation will be required where recovery is only partial or does not occur because the underlying cause proves not to be amenable to treatment.

During recent years there has developed among professionals a greater appreciation of the tremendous contribution family carers make not only to their own elderly person, but also to the community as a whole, and — perhaps more importantly — of the great personal cost involved in so doing. For many families the caring commitment may extend over many years and probably increases as their physical and mental reserves decrease. Where the commitment weighs heavily, unless the carers are comprehensively cared for too, considerable difficulties — physical, emotional and social — may ensue. Since much of the professional help available is directed towards the elderly living alone, this is currently the cause of much concern.

Schemes such as the Home Care Course instituted by Nora Saddington in South Birmingham have proved most successful, not only because of the caring skills they teach, but also because of the opportunities they present to get out and to share problems with others in similar situations. The Association of Carers was begun in 1981, aiming nationally to bring the needs of carers to the attention of policymakers in health and social services departments, and locally to offer practical and social support, with advice on finances, housing, equipment, holidays and the statutory services. Two years after its inception the Association was receiving 22 000 letters annually from carers all over the country, and its compass and influence has extended considerably since (for example, in the campaign to get Invalid Care Allowance paid to married and cohabiting women).

The last decade has seen the recognition and professional acknowledgement of the sad reality of old age abuse — sometimes referred to as non-accidental injury of the elderly or 'granny battering', Christopher Cloke[2] defines this as 'the systematic and continuous abuse of an elderly person by the carer, often, though not always, a relative on whom the elderly person person is dependent for care'. An interesting term is that used by Dr Elizabeth Hocking — 'miscare'. She feels that many families began their caring commitment with genuine concern and sympathy, but that they have been overwhelmed by the task, the relationship thus becoming soured, with resultant harm to the elderly person involved.

Physical and mental suffering may be inflicted upon the victim by direct violence, neglect or exploitation. Nurses, with their close involvement in the personal care of the elderly and the support of their carers, may be the first to uncover or to suspect such problems. Rarely is a censorious attitude to the carer appropriate — he or she is as much in need of help as is the elderly person, and when the situation comes to light, immediate action is necessary for the safety of the latter and the relief of the former.

(b) Sheltered housing

By the beginning of 1980, the housing departments of the local authorities in Great Britain had provided more than 250 000 dwellings in 'grouped housing specifically designed for the elderly and serviced by a resident warden' (DOE Statement 82/69) and housing associations 40 000 more. It is through the safe design of the dwellings and the unobtrusive supervision by the wardens that the schemes aim to maintain the independence of the elderly residents.

No one type of accommodation will suit all needs or all tastes and within a sheltered scheme a variety of dwellings may be found. Bungalows, traditionally regarded by the elderly as particularly suitable, may be available for couples capable of a greater degree of independence in relation to housework and a little gardening. Two storey flats are economical of land and the upper units can be utilised by the more active residents and those who dislike sleeping on the ground floor — lifts may be available. In many schemes there is a preponderance of one bedroom flatlets, each with its own toilet, bath or shower and kitchen facilities, but sharing common room, laundry and possibly a guest room. All the dwellings are connected to the warden's office and flat, in the earlier schemes by a bell, in the newer ones by an audio alarm.

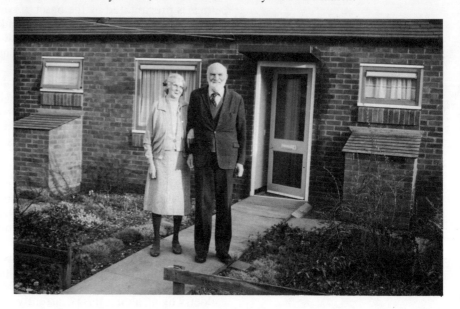

The majority of sheltered schemes consist of approximately 30 units; larger ones have been found to have disadvantages from both a practical and social point of view. It is essential that the elderly are not excluded from the mainstream of life in 'colony' type situations in which segregation and insularity could become inbred. Thus schemes are incorporated within mixed housing developments with ready access to bus stops, shops and other local amenities.

The role of the warden in sheltered schemes is intended to be a supportive and supervisory one; she should not be responsible for domestic assistance or any nursing care that residents may require. The health and social services provision described in the previous chapter is available to sheltered tenants in exactly the same way as it is to other elderly persons in the community.

PAUSE FOR THOUGHT

The success of sheltered housing schemes has been described[3] on the following criteria:

1. Providing old persons with housing specifically designed to take account of their needs, capabilities and limitations.
2. Freeing elderly people from worries such as 'What will happen to me if I am ill, or if I fall?' and giving them greater opportunities to live independently longer in life.
3. Encouraging easy social intercourse with elderly people of similar interests and generally improving the quality of their life . . .

   Can you identify any concern with sheltered schemes?

The major concern with sheltered schemes stems from their very success; people are living within them for much longer than was ever considered likely, and, as the resident's physical or mental health declines, domiciliary services are heavily utilised in order for him to remain in the community. A move at this stage, when the elderly person can least adapt to change, may be seen in human terms as poor management; in any case, a transfer to an elderly persons' home or to a continuing care situation may not be possible because of the considerable demand from elsewhere. Thus the role of the warden in a sheltered scheme is often extended and she assumes considerable responsibility for the more disabled residents' well-being; where this is occurring, it is essential that provision be made for more assistance for her, for more in-service training to equip her more adequately and for more relative help, where available, to be utilised.

Many more sheltered schemes are required to keep pace with demand, and, taking into account the situation described above, some of the units now being planned will be developed as 'very sheltered' schemes (i.e. having several trained wardens and much domiciliary input), while others, such as those run by the Brendoncare Foundation, will incorporate a residential home on the same site into which tenants can move on a temporary or permanent basis if necessary. There are advantages and disadvantages to this idea, which needs to be more thoroughly evaluated in practice before widespread schemes are commissioned.

(c) Residential care

Under Part III of the National Assistance Act 1948 local authorities are required to provide 'residential accommodation for persons who by reason of age, infirmity or any other circumstances are in need of care and attention which is not otherwise available to them'; residential homes so provided have thus tended to be known as 'Part III accommodation'. Since demand has exceeded supply especially in recent years, private residential and nursing homes (the former registered with the local authorities, the latter with the health authorities) have also increased in number and many social services departments are obliged to financially support residents in the private and voluntary schemes to make good their shortfall.

Indeed, the growth of the independent sector has been encouraged by the government policies of the early 1980s, and legislation such as the Nursing Homes and Mental Nursing Homes Act of 1984 has been introduced to tighten up regulations relating to private care. Anxieties have been voiced about the standards of care in some homes, however, and the responsibility placed upon the inspectors to ensure that adequate and appropriate care is given and that staff are effectively trained and utilised must be taken very seriously.

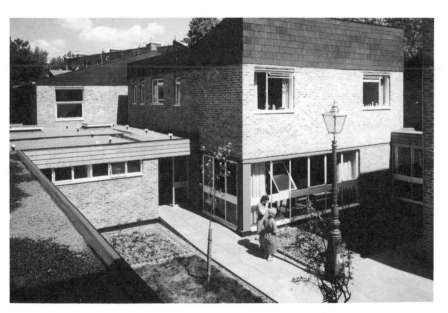

A series of annual censuses of residents living in Part III accommodation has been undertaken by the Joint Unit for Social Services Research at Sheffield University, and these indicate that the type of resident now catered for differs markedly from the type envisaged enjoying the 'residential hotel' facilities described by Aneurin Bevan when the National Assistance bill was presented. Many are physically frail and a proportion mentally confused and thus considerable demands on the care staff exist; in-service training schemes are now more common than they were but are still not widely available for this group.

Admission to residential care is arranged by a social worker and the psychological aspects require at least as much consideration as the practical. Not only is a home given up but also the majority of a person's possessions; he has to adapt his own personal routine and lifestyle to fit in with community life. It is salutary to reflect that there is an increased morbidity and mortality rate in the first six months after relocation to residential care, and even more concerning that recent research has indicated that about a third of admissions could be prevented by supportive input into the person's own home at the time of application, and a further third if intervention had occurred before this.[4]

It must be realised that group living and the presence of staff may in fact be conducive to further dependency unless steps are taken to counter this. The newer homes are designed to encourage privacy and self-sufficiency as far as is possible; there are bedsitting rooms with toilets and showers, and minor catering facilities available to enable the resident to make tea or coffee and light snacks for himself or his visitors. In the older homes, however, residents are more likely to share rooms with one or more others and the resultant lack of privacy and opportunity to be alone as desired may distress some older people greatly.

Improved physical facilities in themselves, however, are not the be all and end all in residential care; it is the attitude of the staff that ultimately confines or liberates the residents. Sensitive assessment of individual need is vital, with care planned around minimum intervention and maximum enhancement of opportunities for self-sufficiency; it should be totally supportive, in no way custodial. Until sufficient numbers of staff appreciative of this concept are recruited, however, many possibilities in residential care will not be realised. 'The residential home is a community facility, it belongs to the people and, above all, to the people who live in it . . . we should start with the residents as the basic managers. Residents must be able to enjoy their personal privacy and decision-making to the very limits of their wishes and capacities;[5] at present perhaps, a counsel of perfection — but an eventual possibility in a so-called democratic society?

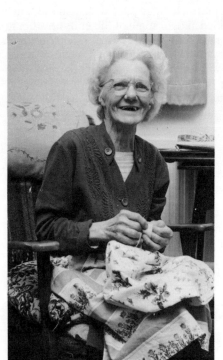

PAUSE FOR THOUGHT

For elderly people seeking admission to homes in the private sector, there may be considerable difficulty in deciding between them unless the facilities and care offered, or lack of them, are made explicit. Can you suggest ways of overcoming this problem?

Concerned about this situation, over a two-year period Liz Day,[6] a specialist Health Visitor, developed with the assistance of colleagues throughout the country a questionnaire for use by elderly people and their families, designed to build up working profiles of homes under consideration. A range of questions covers accommodation, activities within the home, staffing, finances, nursing care available, and policies on visiting and clothing; from the responses obtained, profiles can be built up and an informed choice can then be made. Excerpts from the questionnaire are illustrated opposite. This would seem to be a very sensible approach to the problem, as asking advice from other residents and taking personal recommendations, while useful in themselves, may not highlight areas of particular personal importance to the elderly person concerned.

QUESTIONNAIRE FOR THOSE SEEKING ACCOMMODATION IN OLD PEOPLE'S HOMES/NURSING HOMES/RESIDENTIAL ACCOMMODATION

A. ACCOMMODATION

1. Does the accommodation include: single rooms, double rooms, shared rooms?
2. Does the accommodation provide for married couples?
3. If I share a room with another resident, am I able to meet/interview the prospective resident?
4. If I share a room, and the other resident and I do not hit it off, will I be given the opportunity to change rooms as and when the opportunity arises?
5. Can residents bring their own furniture? If so, what: bed, TV, etc.?
6. Are there communal facilities — e.g. lounge, smoking room, TV room, dining room, etc.?
7. Is there a garden for the use of residents?
8. Can residents share with the gardening?
9. Is there a lift?
10. Do any rooms have their own toilet facilities?
11. How many bathrooms are there?
12. Do any rooms have their own bathrooms?

. . .

B. FINANCES

29. What are the charges per week?
30. Are there any extra charges not included in the weekly rate?
31. Are charges paid weekly or monthly?
32. What day/date are charges to be paid?
33. How often are the charges reviewed?
34. How much warning is given if charges are to change?
35. What would happen if I were to go into hospital and my discharge date were unknown? Would my room be reserved for me at a reduced rate until I was discharged?
36. How long would you keep my room available for me in these circumstances?
37. What would happen if I were to have inadequate financial support to meet the charges?
38. Do residents manage their own financial affairs?

. . .

C. CLOTHING

54. Is there a personal laundry service?
55. Are residents allowed to wear their own clothes?
56. Can residents bring their own bedding/household linen?

References

1. Abrams, M., *Beyond Three Score Years and Ten,* Age Concern, Mitcham, Surrey, 1978
2. Cloke, C., *Old Age Abuse in the Domestic Setting — A Review,* Age Concern, 1983
3. Fox, D., Housing and the elderly. In Hobman, D. (editor), *The Impact of Ageing — Strategies for Cure,* Croom Helm, Chapter 5, 1981
4. Tinker, A., *Staying at Home — Helping Elderly People,* HMSO, 1984
5. Banner, G., Stop talking about the elderly, *New Age,* Spring, 1981
6. Day, L., *Questionnaire for Those Seeking Accommodation in Old People's Homes/Nursing Homes/Residential Accommodation,* Health Visitors' Association, 1985

Further reading

Booth, T. and Berry, S., An overdose of care, *Community Care,* 26 July, 1984

Nissel, M., The family costs of looking after handicapped elderly relatives, *Ageing and Society,* **4,** No. 2, 1984, 185–204

Home Life: A Code of Practice for Residential Care, Centre for Policy on Ageing, 1984

Registration and Inspection of Nursing Homes: A Handbook for Health Authorities, National Association of Health Authorities for England and Wales, 1985

Garrett, G., Old age abuse, *Professional Nurse,* **1,** No. 11, 1986, 304–305

Chapter 9   Hospital provision

In general hospitals at any given time a high proportion of beds in medical and surgical units will be found to contain elderly patients; with the current rise in the numbers of elderly already discussed, the same applies in trauma wards, ophthalmology units, neurological departments — indeed almost every ward with the exception of obstetric and paediatric! In the acute phase of an older person's illness — perhaps appendicitis or strangulation of a hernia – this may well be the most appropriate area in which he should be cared for; but for certain patients, notably the older elderly, in certain instances such a designation is often detrimental to progress.

> **PAUSE FOR THOUGHT**
>
> From your experience working in general medical and surgical areas, can you identify any potential problems for elderly patients who are nursed within them?

Three problems which you may have identified give much cause for concern when elderly patients are cared for within general wards.

The first of these is the emphasis so often placed on the medical condition with which the patient presents to the exclusion (or at least relegation to second place) of other problems which he may be experiencing, which are equally important in the overall perspective. The medical staff are particularly guilty of this; although they are now more appreciative of the diverse physical problems from which the elderly suffer, there is often little realisation that 'multiple pathology' covers functional, mental and social difficulties too — all with an enormous bearing on the outcome of the physical. With the homage paid to individualised care planned following thorough assessment of needs and problems, the nurse should not be an accomplice in this folly of her medical colleagues; that she often is, is a sad reflection on the profession's ability always to practise what it preaches.

A second potential problem is the pace at which a general ward functions. It is often geared to more rapid rehabilitation after illness or surgery than that

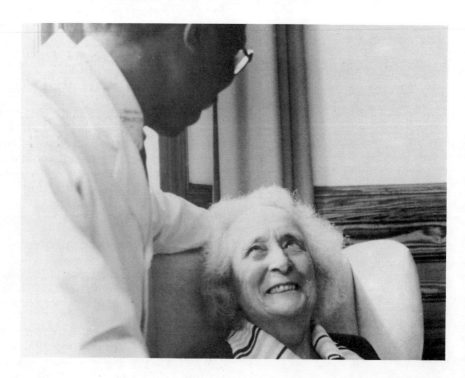

generally achievable in elderly patients, whose recovery and convalescence may be protracted.

The third possible problem often stems from this; the medical staff's 'need for the bed' may mean that discharge is precipitate and may thus not allow for the totality of the patient's situation to be taken into account. Rarely is the elderly patient 'discharged' — leaving hospital almost invariably involves a transfer of his care to community staff or relatives and this cannot be arranged in minutes. A smooth transition from hospital to home care depends on careful preparation of both the patient and his relatives or community personnel; this can only be accomplished with time.

To go some way towards overcoming the problems experienced when an old person is 'stranded' in an acute general ward following surgery or medical illness, it would behove those nurses who are not conversant with the principles of the management of the elderly person's needs to approach their colleagues in the Geriatric Department for advice, initiating a 'nursing consultation'. This tends not to occur on an informal basis very often; the idea could be explored more thoroughly to the benefit of all concerned.

Placing of elderly care beds

PAUSE FOR THOUGHT

What arguments, however, can you identify against caring for elderly people in specialised geriatric units?

The designation of an area as 'geriatric' may in itself be detrimental. The original meaning of the word has become severely adulterated (*see* Part 2, Chapter 7), and it is often now used in a derogatory manner, not only by lay people, but also, sadly, by some professionals. It has been suggested[1] that perhaps our elderly care units need another title less fraught with misunderstandings and encapsulating fewer stereotypical expectations.

Arguments have been advanced that the segregation of elderly people in separate units acts against their best interests in that it relegates them to a 'special' category, 'different' from patients in general areas, and that it thus reinforces negative images of ageing and the elderly. Where units are sited away from acute services and are thereby deprived of facilities such as pathology, X-ray and therapy personnel, the service offered may indeed be inferior and all too often such situations are compounded by unenlightened management 'making do' with a depleted and unimaginative staff.

Perhaps there is nothing wrong in highlighting 'differences', however, if doing so results in positive discrimination and thus enhances care. Children are quite rightly felt to merit care in paediatric units, having 'special' needs not catered for in general wards; ophthalmic patients are cared for in eye units by nurses with a special interest and qualification in their care. A nurse researcher suggests that where elderly patients are nursed in general medical wards they fare badly in competition with patients needing more 'urgent' attention from the nurses.[2]

With these and the points made above in mind, the Geriatric Unit, knowing well the special needs and the potential problems of the elderly sick, can be said to provide 'whole person care'. Being concerned with the clinical, social, preventive and remedial aspects of an older person's illness or disability in a variety of environments, by many it is seen as the most appropriate situation for his hospital stay.

Assessment and rehabilitation

When using the above phrase it is essential to recall that, in nursing terms, it is something of a misnomer. 'Assessment' as a nursing activity takes place wherever patients require the utilisation of nursing skills, and continues to take place in an ongoing manner as long as that need persists, in both hospital and the community. 'Rehabilitation' techniques are not only employed with those recovering from an acute illness or injury; they are also vital to prevent relapse at a later stage, following transfer back into the community or into continuing care facilities. Thus the term has more relevance in a medical sense perhaps than our own.

The vast majority of elderly patients entering geriatric units will do so through assessment and rehabilitation beds; since many will be acutely ill on admission, perhaps following myocardial infarction or cerebrovascular accident, such beds need to be sited within general hospitals with ready access to pathological, X-ray and other facilities. Medical assessment on admission will take account of physical, mental, functional and social ability; only when all four aspects have been thoroughly investigated can realistic plans for rehabilitation be formulated by the patient and staff together. In the early days of care in such a unit there will be a high level of nursing and therapeutic input; this support will gradually be withdrawn as the patient progresses. For the proportion of patients whose underlying condition is found to preclude improvement, however, sustained support until the natural conclusion is required.

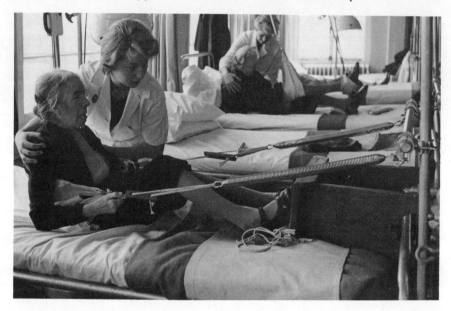

Approximately 50% of the patients admitted to assessment and rehabilitation beds will be discharged back into the community, to their own homes and families, within three months. Twenty-five per cent will not recover from the conditions which necessitated their admissions; they will die within two months of admission. The remaining 25% will not recover sufficiently either to return unaided to the community or to be supported by family or friends where these exist; they are the people for whom residential facilities or continuing care in hospital will be required.

Continuing care

Where ongoing physical or mental disability means that a patient cannot return home or to community care, placement for continuing care must be considered. The philosophy of cure gives way to that of care and the realistic aim becomes the maintenance of the individual at his maximum level of functioning in the situation.

PAUSE FOR THOUGHT

For many elderly patients a continuing care unit will be the last home they will know; as such, a 'home' it should be. As a nurse manager on a planning team working on a purpose-built unit, what would you consider important with respect to (a) its siting and design, and (b) the facilities offered?

Perhaps this activity was seen as unrealistic in view of the fact that most nurses work in continuing care units that were anything but purpose-built; all too often they were converted from the remains of the workhouse or salvaged from the dissolution of the tuberculosis or infectious diseases unit. Also no indication was given of the financial or other constraints which inevitably exist to dog any new venture!

However, if the ideal can be identified, it is possible to work towards it within the bounds of realism. Not all improvements are dependent upon a large increase in finances; many, especially in relation to improving the quality of life of the elderly, are intimately tied up with staff attitudes. The latter, sadly, are frequently harder to alter than the budgets.

As their advocate, it is the hopes and wishes of elderly people themselves that the nurse should put forward in planning for their care; it is their perception of their needs and problems which is of the utmost importance. The danger of making blanket assumptions with regard to the elderly has already been described; few would question, however, the view so forcibly put by Mary Stott,[3] columnist and writer, now in her 80s: 'It is not "right" for us to have to share a bedroom with four strangers, or a lounge with 40. It is not "right" for us to be stranded miles away from family, friends and associates in geriatric wards. It is not "right" for most of us to be segregated by age from the rest of the community. The "right" way for most of us to live is the way we have always lived, in a mixed-sex, mixed-age community.'

How, then, for a continuing care setting can the nurse assist in planning as 'normal' an environment as possible? Firstly, with regard to siting; while an out-of-town, country location may sound idyllic, from a practical viewpoint — residents being able to integrate with the local community, families maintaining contact, staff getting to work — it is totally unsuitable. The unit needs to be sited near a centre where there can be ready access to parks, pubs, shops and churches — the usual gathering places of everyday life. The mixed age community advocated by Mary Stott can be achieved by the integration of a young chronic sick unit on the same site; since many of the facilities provided for the one — physiotherapy, diversional therapy, social support — will be required by the other, it is a sound economic as well as humane grouping.

Single-storey design allows for a greater degree of independence for residents able to use the gardens and outside facilities; adequate space is essential to allow for the passage of wheelchairs, walking frames and other aids, especially in areas with a lot of furniture, such as dining annexes. Where ward units are composed of single or double rooms, not only are the residents able to enjoy more privacy but also, as the ward can cater for both sexes, beds may be more readily available for admissions as required. Another vitally important point is that partners can remain together in this situation. Central facilities for large group functions should supplement the individual dining and recreation areas in each ward. Easily accessible toilets, with adaptations as required, are essential in all areas used by the residents and not simply the wards.

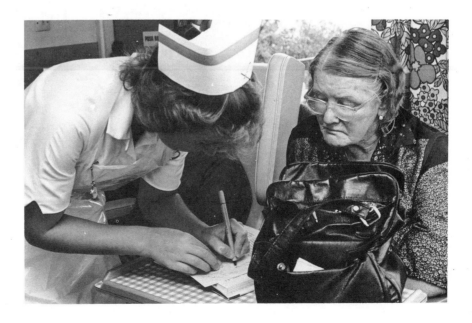

A universal need is a degree of personal space in which to be oneself; where it is not possible for residents to have individual rooms or cubicles, judicious siting of furniture, with chests of drawers or wardrobes acting as dividers, can to some degree fulfil this need. The furnishings within the unit need to be homely and non-clinical; safety and fire precautions obviously have to be heeded but where personal preferences of residents can be permitted they should be. Is there any reason why the elderly woman should not have her own curtains at the window or her own counterpane on her bed?

Personal bedding and clothing require rather different laundry facilities from those usually serving hospital wards. Individual automatic washing machines with tumble driers in the ward areas not only overcome the problems of delay and loss in a centralised laundry but also offer the opportunity to involve residents in the care of their own property.

Library, hairdressing, shop and chapel facilities need to be present on site for residents unable to leave the unit; how much more 'normal', however, for them to be able to visit the local library, salon, store or church wherever possible. The cry that there are insufficient staff available to enable residents to do this is invalidated where relatives, friends and community volunteers can perform this service for them. Good links with local groups are essential in continuing care work; in most areas there is still a vast untapped source of goodwill and practical help in schools, colleges, church congregations, women's groups and retirement clubs.

Community volunteers can be of immeasurable help in the provision of recreational and educational facilities for elderly residents. Radio, television and weekly bingo, while all having their valid uses, can hardly be said to meet optimally the needs of the majority of residents; each person's interests need to be sensitively assessed on admission and assistance planned to enable him to continue as far as he is able with them. An elderly man admitted to a local continuing care unit had not in 30 years missed a home game of Bristol City; his life now revolves around the weekly visits of another young fan, who brings in news of the team and detailed descriptions of their victories (their recent series of defeats he has tended to gloss over!). Until her severe stroke, an elderly woman in the same unit had been a regular attender at the Sisterhood meetings at the local Baptist chapel; the organisation of volunteer transport enabled her to maintain weekly contact with her old friends and lifestyle throughout the two years she spent in continuing care before her death.

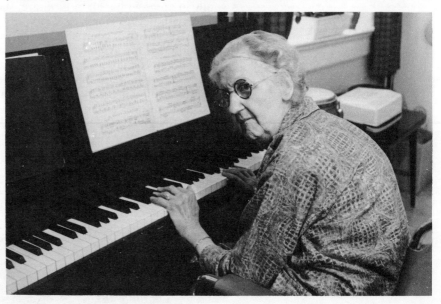

Day hospitals

A day hospital has been defined[4] as '. . . a building to which patients may come or be brought in the morning, where they spend several hours in therapeutic activity and from whence they return subsequently on the same day to their own homes' — it provides 'office hours' hospital care including medical and nursing treatment, speech therapy, occupational therapy and physiotherapy, chiropody and hairdressing.

PAUSE FOR THOUGHT

Can you identify some of the advantages of day hospital care to the patient and his family from the following brief case study?

Albert Franks, a 76-year-old man who lived at home with his 74-year-old wife and their 32-year-old daughter (who suffers from Down's syndrome), was admitted to hospital following a cerebrovascular accident. He had a right-sided paralysis and marked speech difficulty. At first his progress was slow, but six weeks after admission he was ambulant with the aid of a tripod and could communicate sufficiently to make his needs understood. He was, however, very depressed and the decision was made to allow him to go home, with domiciliary nursing support and visits to the day hospital three times weekly for speech therapy, occupational therapy and physiotherapy.

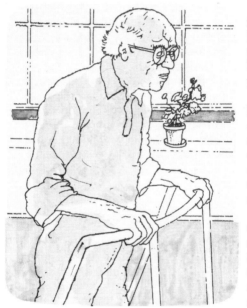

Firstly, the availability of day hospital care enabled Mr Franks to be transferred back into the community at a much earlier stage than would otherwise have been possible; there was little chance of regression following his initial progress as remedial therapy was to continue on a regular basis. Prolonged hospitalisation with its attendant dangers of depression and dependency in the patient, anxiety and separation for the family could thus be avoided.

It must not be forgotten, however, that the care of another after a recent illness is often demanding and wearing on an elderly person; the situation described in the case study was exacerbated by Mrs Franks's need to care also for her handicapped daughter. She, in fact, was at a training centre during the week; consequently the three days on which her husband attended the day hospital provided Mrs Franks with short breaks in which she could relax and also keep up outside social contacts; without these breaks she may well not have been able to cope.

Other advantages of day hospital care include the fact that it may obviate the need for in-patient care entirely when an elderly patient can be investigated and treated on an out-patient basis, thus avoiding the trauma of admission. The anaemic patient, for example, may have blood tests, electrocardiograms and sternal marrow puncture carried out in the unit; samples of excreta can be obtained for testing on the same visit. On subsequent visits, when the type and the cause of the anaemia have been ascertained, the appropriate therapy can be given.

A day hospital also supplements in-patient facilities and, when it is sited in a district general hospital, wards other than those of the geriatric unit (medical, orthopaedic) may also utilise its personnel and their expertise. Prior to discharge, patients from the ward areas can be introduced to the day hospital and its staff; fears may be alleviated and the transition made easier when the continuity of care is demonstrated by the same people dealing with the patients before and after discharge.

Day hospital care is not appropriate when the Primary Health Care Team could cope satisfactorily with the patient and family's needs; in the care study above, Mr Franks was in fact receiving domiciliary nursing but the remedial aspects of his care could only adequately be undertaken in the day hospital environment. Nor is day hospital care appropriate when needs are primarily social; certainly the social aspects of day hospital care are important in re-integration following illness or disability, and in boosting morale, but unless medical, nursing or remedial input is also required, referral for Day Centre placement should be made.

The facilities described here — day hospitals, assessment and rehabilitation and continuing care — are now common to most geriatric units throughout the country; for description of the hospital facilities available for the elderly with psychiatric disorders, the reader is referred to *Care of the Mentally Ill*, by Peggy Martin, another part of the Essentials of Nursing course. To complete the picture of hospital provision, however, it is necessary to mention briefly certain experimental schemes currently being implemented.

Other provision

(a) Five-day wards

Wards which admit elderly patients from Monday to Friday can provide more intensive rehabilitation programmes than those available in day hospitals; sometimes they enable care to be more effectively shared between hospital and family.

(b) Hospital-at-home schemes

These are more common in parts of Europe but have been developed in some areas in this country. The same staff, both nursing and remedial, are available in both the hospital and the community to ease the crucial period of transition from hospital to home care.

(c) National Health Service nursing homes

Three experimental schemes have been set up between District Health Authorities and the Department of Health and Social Security to open units giving nursing home style care within the National Health Service, in accord with recommendations made in paragraphs 8.23–8.37 of *Growing Older* (Cmnd 8173). The units, accommodating between 20 and 30 residents, opened in Portsmouth, Sheffield and Fleetwood during 1983 and 1984, and are intended to provide for elderly people not able to benefit from further medical treatment or rehabilitation, and needing continuous, long-term nursing care. Stressing domesticity and the allowance to the residents of as much autonomy as possible, they offer the ideal opportunity to change the emphasis in care from a medical to a truly nursing model.

Over the five-year period of the experiment the health of the residents, and their views and those of the staff about the care provided and the costs of the system, are being evaluated by a team from the University of Newcastle upon Tyne. Several Health Authorities, however, are already planning to set up their own Homes on the same principles, and this has wide implications for the organisation of services for elderly people in the decades to come.

Liaison between hospital and community

It must be remembered that for the vast majority of elderly people a stay in hospital means only a short interlude in their life as a whole; they come into hospital from their own homes and/or family care and return to them after treatment. The transition from one environment to the other has been recognised of late to be of vital importance; research has indicated that insufficient attention is paid to it, especially with regard to discharge procedures: 'Discharge from hospital is often a badly planned process and sometimes can hardly be described as planned at all'.[5]

Ward staff must be conversant with the elderly person's home situation and care network as appropriate. The active involvement of relevant community nursing staff when discharge plans are made — and they should tentatively be made as early as possible during hospitalisation — is vital. A variety of structured forms have evolved to travel with the patient as a means of conveying care plans; while the design used depends on local needs and preferences, an essential feature is the name and designation of the referring nurse so that ready contact can be made if necessary after discharge.

A frequent problem for ward staff, even when using a problem-oriented approach to patient care, is the difficulty of evaluating discharge planning outcome; the patient leaves the ward and effectively the remit of the staff in it. Sadly, feedback may only reach the staff if readmission becomes necessary or complaints are channelled back through community staff. Where a community liaison worker exists, this problem is considerably lessened; by regularly reporting back at joint meetings on the progress of individual patients, the community worker enables the ward nurse to see the value of her longer-term care planning and thus to continue with and improve her practice in the future.

References

1. Brocklehurst, J.C., What's in a name? *New Age*, **24,** No. 28, 1984
2. Fielding, P., *An Examination of Student Nurses' Attitudes towards Older People in Hospital,* Royal College of Nursing, 1986
3. Stott, M., *Ageing for Beginners*, Blackwell, p. 48, 1981
4. Brocklehurst, J., *The Geriatric Day Hospital,* King Edward's Hospital Fund for London, p. 11, 1970
5. Turton, P. and Wilson Barnett, J., Nursing services. In Simpson, P.J.E. and Levitt, R. (editors), *Going Home: A Guide for Helping the Patient on Leaving Hospital*, Churchill Livingstone, p. 265, 1981

Further reading

The Experimental National Health Service Nursing Homes for Elderly People — An Outline, DHSS, April, 1985

Garrett, G., Sharing the caring — the hospital and the community in the care of the elderly, *Professional Nurse*, **1**, No. 1, 1985, 19–20

Martin, P., *Care of the Mentally Ill,* Macmillan, 1987

Chapter 10   Nursing approach

As in any other branch of nursing, in the care of the elderly the unique function of the nurse is 'assisting the individual (sick or well) in the performance of those activities contributing to health or its recovery, or to a peaceful death, that he would perform unaided if he had the necessary strength, will or knowledge'.[1] The aspects of individualised care of especial importance in respect of elderly persons are discussed in Part 4 of this book; there are, however, five vitally important concepts in caring for the elderly generally and these will be outlined and discussed here. They are the preservation of dignity and individuality, the promotion of effective communication, the encouragement of self-care, the education of the patient and his family and multi-disciplinary teamwork.

Preservation of dignity and individuality

Aspects of this topic have already been covered from the community care position in Chapter 7. Perhaps the reader will look again at the opening paragraphs of that chapter and recall how the elderly in the community can be assisted in maintaining these attributes.

The admission of the elderly patient to hospital is frequently associated with:

1. The loss of the ability to manage one's own physical needs (washing, dressing, toileting, feeding).
2. The loss of the ability to fulfil one's psychological needs (security, status, social interaction).
3. The need to conform (with limitation of choice in everyday matters, the pursuit of individual interests).

Because of the nature of the experience, some adaptation is inevitably required of the elderly patient but the aim should be to minimise the effects of the losses and to maximise the patient's potential within it.

PAUSE FOR THOUGHT

It is sometimes a salutary experience to look critically at our own ward areas; do so at your own over a span of duty. How conducive is the environment to the maintenance of the patient's dignity and individuality? What evidence is there of a positive staff attitude in this respect?

You may perhaps have devised a check-list against which facilities and attitudes could be gauged; items on it could include the following:

- How much privacy is afforded to the patient?
- Are there effective curtains around the bedspace?
- Are these used correctly by all staff when exposure could compromise the patient's dignity?
- Is the patient exposed as little as possible during examinations and nursing procedures?
- Is there a separate secluded area which can be used (a) by staff to interview patients and (b) by patients wishing to discuss personal matters (e.g. with relatives or social workers)?
- Are there locks on lavatory and bathroom doors (with adequate safety aids and call bells at hand)?
- When the patient needs supervision of toileting or bathing, is this done discreetly and unobtrusively?
- Are 'accidents', incontinence and communication difficulties dealt with promptly in a sympathetic but professional manner?

- What evidence is there of respect of individuality?
- If the patient is in bed, is he in his own night wear?
- If the patient is up, is he wearing his own day clothes?
- Is the patient referred to by his/her correct title (Mr Jones/Miss Blythe)?
- Is the patient's opinion sought in conversations with staff?
- Is there 'evidence' of 'home' about — cut flowers from a garden, photographs on the locker?
- Are lockers sufficiently large to accommodate clothing and personal possessions?
- Where a menu system is in operation, does the patient select his own meals?
- Is the patient able to involve himself in ward activities of his own choice? Can he opt out of those that are not of his choosing?
- Is the radio or television tuned to the channel of the patient's choice?
- Within the limits of his condition, is the patient free to get up, to retire, to take a rest on his bed when he chooses?

This is by no means an exclusive list and you may well have considered many other points. Certainly many wards do not have optimum facilities but the environment can generally be manipulated with little, if any, financial outlay in this respect. In the final analysis, it is the attitude of the staff exemplified by their behaviour which preserves or destroys the vital human qualities of dignity and individuality in the elderly patients for whom they care.

Promotion of effective communication

PAUSE FOR THOUGHT

What factors are important in ensuring effective communication? Why may some elderly people experience problems with these?

For effective communication to occur, a 'message' from one person has to be transmitted to another and understood by that second person in the manner in which it was intended by the first. Although verbal messages (i.e. the spoken word) are often considered to be the main channel of communication in our society, equally — if not more — important are the non-verbal channels by which we express ourselves (facial expression, eye contact, gesture, posture, body contact and the use of space).

If verbal communication is to be effective, speech and hearing mechanisms have to be intact and functional, and these include the relevant brain centres and pathways as well as the actual respiratory, oral and auditory equipment for the generation and reception of sound. The language used has to be that understood by the receiving person. That person needs to be able to see the communicator to be able to pick up non-verbal signals and to have intact touch perception to appreciate body contact. Unless there is free body movement, the ability to express oneself in gesture and posture and in using the space around is impoverished.

Elderly people may experience difficulty with communication for a variety of reasons. Failing eyesight and hearing are common causes — some 60% of the over 70s are deaf to some degree — and physical and social problems may make for difficulties in obtaining and using aids to overcome these disabilities, and also in maintaining them thereafter. Speech difficulties — both expressive and receptive ones — may follow stroke and other cerebral disorders, such as Parkinsonism. The former may also affect reading and writing ability, and sensory and movement deficits may also inhibit non-verbal communication.

In a broad sense social and emotional factors must also be considered. Major upheavals in lifestyle, such as a bereavement or the loss of a home through relocation, may have adverse effects on the will and the ability to socialise; if the person feels for some reason socially unacceptable (for example, because of incontinence), there may be withdrawal and isolation. If he is isolated for any length of time, the elderly person may then simply lose the skill of social communication.

To promote effective communication with elderly patients, the nurse must become proficient at sensitive assessment (see next chapter) and be able to intervene appropriately to assist with overcoming any highlighted problems. Such intervention may range from simple measures such as siting herself appropriately when talking to the hearing-impaired patient (in good lighting, at face level, in reasonably close proximity), to the use of sophisticated equipment such as electronic communicators. However, it is not possible fully to do justice to so important an aspect of the nursing approach to elderly people in this chapter, and the reader is referred to the further reading sources suggested at its end.

Self-care

The art of geriatric nursing has been defined as 'the enlightened withdrawal of support'; while perhaps a somewhat simplistic definition in some ways, this is certainly one very important aspect of the care of the elderly which merits some consideration here.

In hospital or community the initial assessment of the elderly patient will identify his capabilities and examine his limitations in relation to direct personal care (toileting, washing, dressing, feeding) and extended personal care (shopping, cooking, housework, socialising). Care will be planned accordingly to strengthen his capabilities and to lessen his limitations. Constant review of the situation is required to ensure that care continues to be appropriate to need — to check that assistance is no longer being provided for an activity that the patient can now manage unaided or, alternatively, that no new difficulty has arisen for which help is required.

Difficulties in the promotion of self-care can be anticipated from both the patient's and the carer's perspective. The patient may adopt the dependent role if encouraged to do so, abandoning attempts to recover self-caring capacities. Relatives — and, not infrequently, nurses — find great difficulty in standing back and watching as shaving is painstakingly undertaken or clothing laboriously donned; they frequently intervene prematurely and thus rob the elderly patient of his triumph at succeeding unaided. However limited the degree of independence achieved, it reinforces for the individual his sense of self-worth; this should be remembered in continuing care settings where the encouragement of self-care is as vital as in the home or the rehabilitation unit.

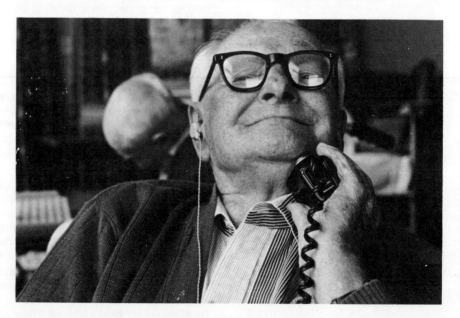

The well-motivated patient may overcome considerable handicaps to become self-caring. The setting of realistic goals assists motivation, and encouragement and praise reinforce success. More difficulty of course is experienced with the poorly motivated patient; he should not be labelled as uncooperative, but rather every effort should be made to find out why he lacks the drive to participate more fully in his care. There may be underlying medical reasons such as depression (a feature of many disorders such as Parkinsonism, or — understandably — a sequel to disabling illnesses such as stroke), infection or incipient heart failure. Perhaps where losses of supports or faculties preceded illness, there may seem little left to get better for; if return to an unsatisfactory home situation is foreseen after hospitalisation, little effort may be made to hasten it. Only when such problems are identified and discussed can steps be taken towards their solution — and motivation hopefully engendered.

Self-care can only be reasonably encouraged in an environment with which the patient is familiar and in which he feels confident. This is obviously less likely to be a problem for the patient cared for at home, in his own surroundings, although adaptations to these may be necessary to overcome the effects of disability (for example, the provision of a raised toilet seat or a support rail by the bath). In ward areas safety precautions are vital to protect the self-caring patient and these include ensuring that beds and chairs are of the correct height, that walking aids are checked and in good order and that adequate lighting is available (in requisite areas by night as well as by day). Individual limitations to self-care (which will be discussed in more detail in Part 4) may often be overcome by relatively simple means: for the patient with urgency, by siting her bed at the end of the ward, close to the toilet; for the hemiplegic, facilitating dressing and undressing by the provision of Velcro fastenings on trousers and shirts; and for the arthritic, adapting cutlery to permit independent feeding.

To return briefly to the quotation which opened this section of the chapter, the key word in it could be seen to be 'enlightened'. Withdrawal of support for the elderly rarely occurs as a constant tail-off over a period of time; appropriate responses must be made following sensitive assessment of the patient's fluctuating needs. For example, tiredness or irritability may retard the dressing efforts of the hemiplegic patient who, to date, has done well; if frustration and consequent demoralisation are not to be experienced, unobtrusive assistance must be given. This should not be seen as encouraging dependency but rather as maintaining (indirectly) his independence.

It must be pointed out in concluding this section that, even when all possible safety precautions have been taken, the encouragement of self-care for the elderly and disabled inevitably involves a degree of risk-taking. In their own homes the elderly constantly run risks and these are generally accepted as justifiable by those caring for them; indeed, patients are taught how to get up unaided after a fall, how to summon help if necessary. In hospital we are reluctant to allow any chance of an 'incident' with its attendant enquiries and documentation, recriminations from anxious relatives or senior staff; anxiety about the latter may inhibit the promotion of the maximum degree of self-care possible. Thus it is vital that, where appropriate, relatives be involved in the planning of care and appreciate the principles underlying it. Equally vital is the assurance from senior staff that, where there is adherence to all required safety regulations, every support will be given to ward staff in their attempts to encourage self-care to the benefit of their elderly patients.

Education of the patient and his family

The general features of health education for the elderly were also considered in Chapter 8. The following paragraphs will concentrate on the practical aspects of promoting knowledge concerning health and adaptation to disability, teaching basic skills and encouraging positive attitudes.

Community nurses have always accepted and often considerably developed their role as teachers of both patients and their families in acute episodes of illness and in ongoing situations. In comparison, perhaps little emphasis has been placed on the nurse's teaching role in hospital ward or clinic; efforts must be made to prepare nurses more effectively for this as they often bear great responsibility for preparing elderly patients and their relatives for management of continuing disability consequent upon major surgery (such as the formation of a colostomy) or the onset of conditions such as diabetes and stroke.

The first move in the teaching strategy should be the assessment of the readiness to learn. The patient needs to have begun to come to terms with ongoing disability in order to learn how to cope most effectively with it. Some patients never truly do (such as 'Mrs Brown' in the Pause for Thought at the beginning of the second part of Chapter 7); they require continuing support and supervision of treatment. Most elderly patients do adjust, however, but for many this takes time, especially when there is altered body image or changed social status. Relatives may be tired and anxious after a long period of caring or a time of great stress and may not be immediately amenable to learning new skills. Coping with a stoma or giving injections is simply not possible for some people, and nurses should not necessarily expect relatives to carry out these procedures for their elderly nor should they judge their supportive commitment to them only in terms of their ability or otherwise to do so.

A second consideration is how much the patient or his relatives are capable of learning. Obvious factors here include educational status, interest in the problem and the effect of any intellectual deficit that may have occurred with illness. The presence of other conditions may limit what can physically be done: a patient with arthritis or a residual hemiplegia from a previous stroke, for example, may have difficulty managing prostheses unaided; the 62-year-old daughter of the 80-year-old diabetic may herself have poor vision and therefore be unable to draw up accurately her mother's insulin.

Not infrequently nurses feel that they need to teach their unfortunate learners all that they themselves know about a condition! How much is it necessary to teach the patient about his pacemaker or his stoma, his arthritis or his anaemia? Basically, he must be taught sufficient for him to deal safely and confidently with his disability in the home situation. There are those who will want to find out more — perhaps much more — and there are those who will be satisfied with this amount. Further information can be given at a later stage where desired or appropriate but with elderly patients initially the basic practicalities are the most important concern, and ensuring an adequate grasp of these should be the prime objective.

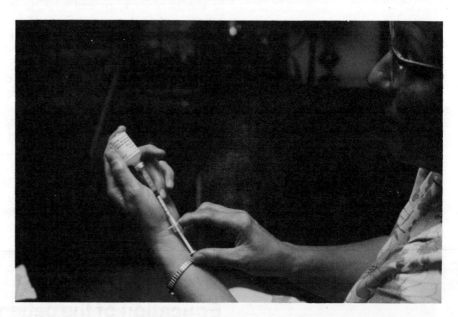

A useful opening move with both patients and relatives is to ascertain their previous knowledge of the condition and its treatment; misconceptions may thus be discovered and fears identified from the start. Memories of 'Aunt Alice', who, after her stroke, 'couldn't do anything for herself ever again', will obviously colour present expectations; 'They have a bag on their front, don't they?' may indicate the limit of the lay person's concept of life for a colostomist. Treatment for many conditions has only become available in recent years, and, not appreciating new advances, the elderly may give themselves poor prognoses.

Having ascertained what is known, the nurse can then work towards the unknown, giving very basic explanations of problems and the effects of treatment: 'Your body hasn't been making enough insulin to help you use sugar; the tablets will encourage it to make more'; 'The opening has taken over the work of your back passage so now you pass your motions into this bag'. Any diagrams, leaflets or other aids used to assist explanation should be sufficiently large to be easily seen and read; they should contain straightforward terms which are readily understood by the patient and his relatives. Home-produced aids, tailored to meet the needs of individuals, are thus often more useful than ready-made commercial ones.

Practical skills (such as testing urine, changing appliances, drawing up and giving injections) are best taught by demonstration with accompanying explanation. The patient or his relatives should be encouraged to handle the equipment, to become familiar with it, to voice any queries about it. Supervised practice with repetition of instructions and prompting as necessary is often required over a period of time before a reasonable degree of confidence and competence is achieved. Praise reinforces success and should be used as liberally as possible; parts of a procedure with which difficulty is experienced should be played down in comparison but then worked on more stringently in the next practice session. Questioning is used to provide feedback where demonstration alone cannot satisfy the nurse that a certain point has been sufficiently understood.

To quote the old adage, 'Attitudes are caught and not taught'; the nurse has a great responsibility to promote positive attitudes to health in ageing and the management of disability. She can only do so when she herself holds these attitudes, however!

Multi-disciplinary teamwork

The members of the Primary Health Care Team and their contributions to the care of the elderly in the community were discussed earlier, in the second part of Chapter 8, and the reader may wish to refer back to this section and recall the points made. In the hospital situation care is also based on a multi-disciplinary approach and this will be considered further here.

PAUSE FOR THOUGHT

Sit in on a team meeting in either a ward or day hospital. From your experience of the meeting:

1. Identify the personnel involved.
2. Discuss their roles in relation to patient care.
3. Note any problems which you think could arise with multi-disciplinary teamwork.

Parts 1 and 2 could have been answered in diagrammatic form as demonstrated in Figure 10.1; the patient ('the centre of our universe, around whom all our works revolve, towards whom all our efforts trend', J.B. Murphy) receives care and support from the personnel named in the inner ring; their roles are clarified in the outer. At the meeting at which you are present some of these may have been absent and others — audiologists, psychologists — may have been seen. For the most part, however, these are the ones figuring most prominently in the team for most patients. You may have found community nurses as well as ward staff attending, a feature of team meetings much encouraged; personal contact can be made with the patient prior to discharge and appropriate follow-up arranged to ensure continuity of care.

One obvious problem which you may have identified is the potential confusion for the patient when many professionals are dealing with his care! The nurse he generally recognises because of her uniform and her constant presence; the occupational therapists and physiotherapists look remarkably alike, however, in tunics and trousers, and doctors, speech therapists, dieticians and chiropodists all wear white coats and may have little to differentiate between them. Each team member should extend to the patient the courtesy of an introduction and an explanation of his role in care; where this is done and all care can be seen by the patient to be part of a concerted whole (i.e. there are common goals to which all personnel are working) confusion is lessened and cooperation more readily achieved.

For the team to function efficiently to the benefit of the patient, each member must be sure of his own position in it and conversant with the roles of the others. Case notes should be kept in common so that there is general

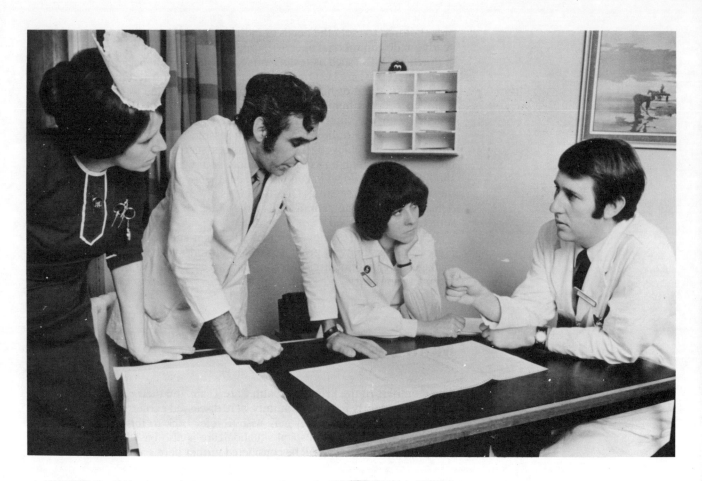

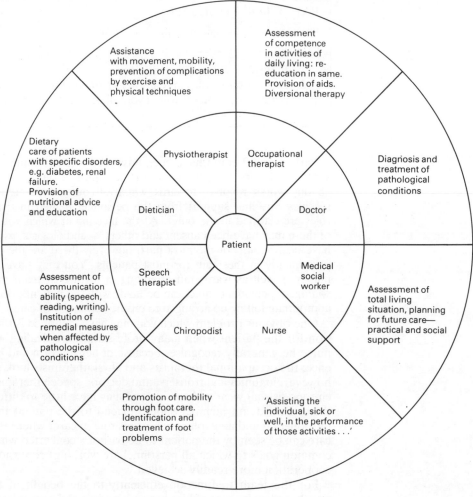

Figure 10.1 The multi-disciplinary team caring for the elderly

awareness of what is happening to a patient and what other input is being made in between team meetings.

The leadership of the team will depend on the principal needs of the different patients — and thus will change with changing needs for the individual patient. For example, the doctor will lead the team caring for the acutely ill elderly patient admitted with left ventricular failure, requiring immediate investigation and resuscitative measures; the occupational therapist may play the principal role in the rehabilitation of the patient with rheumatoid arthritis; the nurse will direct the care for the dying patient and his family. There is no room in the team for professional jealousies or superiorities; only in a trusting, open relationship with respect for one another's professional expertise can it hope to serve the patient effectively.

Reference

1. Henderson, V., *Basic Principles of Nursing Care,* International Council of Nurses, 1960

Further reading

Levene, B., Sensory loss in the elderly, *Nursing*, **2,** No. 41, 1985, 1221–1225

Mcleod Clark, J., Communicating with elderly people. In Redfern, S. (editor), *Nursing Elderly People*, Churchill Livingstone, Chapter 4, 1986

Evers, H., Professional practice and patient care: multidisciplinary teamwork in geriatric wards, *Ageing and Society*, **2,** 1982, 57–75

Part 4   Individualised Care

Chapter 11   Nursing process

Over the last five years considerable interest has been expressed in the use of different nursing models as bases on which to plan, implement and develop care for patients both in hospital and in the community. In some geriatric units the Activities of Living model, developed by Roper, Logan and Tierney, is felt to be the most appropriate; in some, Orem's Self-Care model. Other units use an amalgam of these and others, but many are struggling at present to decide on a philosophical base from which their practical care of elderly patients can realistically emanate. The paragraphs that follow are intended only to discuss the main factors inherent in a nursing process approach, and give no direct allegiance to any particular model; the reader is advised to read again *The Essentials of Nursing: An Introduction*,[1] Chapter 1, and to consult the other texts listed in the Further Reading at the end of this chapter for a full consideration of this very important subject area.

> **PAUSE FOR THOUGHT**
>
> Recall the four stages of the Nursing Process.
>
> Using the information from Chapters 2, 3 and 4 of Part 1 and your own experience, outline any particular points in relation to each stage that you would consider important with elderly clients/patients.

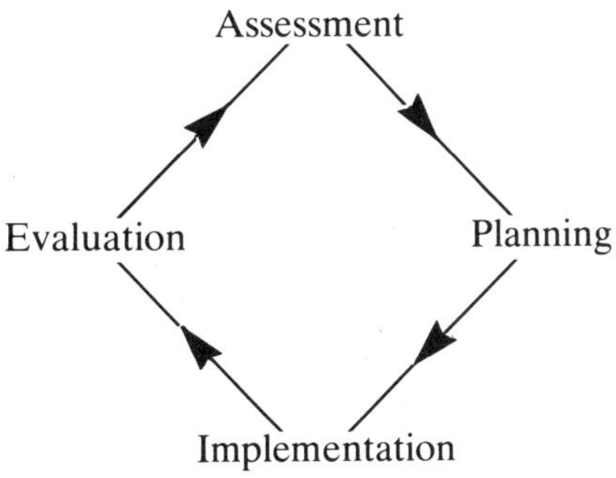

The four stages in the Nursing Process are shown in Figure 11.1. They are demonstrated here in this fashion to underline the fact that they are more dynamic parts of an ongoing whole rather than serial stages with a clear-cut beginning and end.

Figure 11.1   The four stages in the Nursing Process

Assessment

Clearly the ideal place in which to make an assessment of the elderly patient is in his own home and the community nurse has the advantage of being able to do so; she is able to meet him on his own terms as it were, in the situation in which he is usually his most confident, competent self. His capabilities and limitations in his everyday setting can be observed at first hand, his interaction with others in the household can be assessed and problems which are primarily environmental can be noted.

Other than in emergencies, where admission to hospital is required, a member of the medical staff frequently makes a domiciliary visit to aid his assessment and whenever possible a nurse should accompany him to begin hers. Where this is not possible but the patient has been receiving community nursing support, consultation with his community nurse may fill in important gaps in background knowledge.

While a certain amount of personal information is necessary on the admission of any patient to hospital, a detailed interview to obtain a nursing history straight after the admission of an elderly patient may not be appropriate. The patient may be very ill on admission or tired and anxious on having to leave his home for a new and perhaps worrying environment. Relatives or friends accompanying him may provide initial information in this situation; the remainder may be obtained over the next few days as he settles into the ward and becomes more familiar with it. Equally, the first visit made to the patient by the community nurse is unlikely to provide a completely comprehensive picture and information will be added to the history as subsequent visits are made.

Example 1

The history sheet shown in Table 11.1 for Mrs Nancy Norman illustrates how limited information may be initially when a patient is admitted who is very ill. The only available details were obtained from the warden of her sheltered accommodation, who had come in the ambulance with her. Additional information was obtained when Mrs Norman's daughter was contacted and came in but a complete assessment could only be made when she regained full consciousness some days later.

On admission, her priority needs and problems were identified by observation of her physical condition.

Table 11.1   Example 1

NURSING HISTORY AND ASSESSMENT SHEET

Record No. ___022343___

PATIENT LABEL

Mr/Mrs/Miss ___Nancy Norman___

Address ___Flat 6, "Grey Stones,"___
___Britton Road.___
___Bristol.___

Male/Female   Age ___76___

Date of Birth ___12·01·11___

Date of admission/first visit
___06·02·87___

Time ___14·15___

Type: ☐ Routine   ☑ Emergency

    Transfer from: _____

Religion ___None___

Practising/baptised _____

Minister _____

Telephone number _____

Next of kin (name) ___Mrs J. Moore___

Relationship to patient ___Daughter___

Address ___11 Penrith Drive___
___Parkway, Bristol___

Telephone numbers ___621035 (not yet aware NB)___

Contact at night/in emergency   YES/NO

Occupation (or father) ___Retired Housewife___

Marital status ___Widow___

Children (or place in family) ___Daughter (?son abroad)___

Other dependants _____

Pets _____

School (children only) _____

Hobbies _____

Clubs _____

Favourite pastime _____

Does patient smoke?   YES/NO

Speech difficulty/language barrier
___Patient unconscious___

Dysphasia   Dysarthria

Accommodation

Lives alone   YES/NO

Part III/EMI/Old People's Home/Rented

Other ___Warden controlled flatlet for last___
___three months.___

Consultant ___Dr Lloyd___

House officer ___Dr Smith___

Presenting condition _____
___Cerebrovascular accident___

History of present complaint and reason for admission
___Found on living room floor___
___by warden - unconscious___

Past medical history
___Previous small stroke 2 years ago -___
___(left side) good functional___
___recovery___

Allergies

Current medication
___?"blood pressure tablets"___

What patient says is the reason for admission and attitude to admission

Patient's expectations

Any problems at home while/because patient is in hospital?

Relevant home conditions (e.g. stairs)
___First floor flat (2 flights stairs)___

Visiting problems

Care at home

Community nurse _____

No. _____

Name of GP _____ *Dr Reynolds* _____

Address _____ *Dulton Health Centre* _____

Other services involved

Home help _____ Day hospital _____

Laundry _____ Day centre/club _____

Inco supplies _____ Health visitor _____

Aids _____ Social worker _____

Meals on wheels _____ Voluntary worker _____

Daily living

Diet

Special _____

Food or drink dislikes _____

Appetite: ☐ GOOD ☐ POOR

Remarks _____

Sleep

How many hours normally? _____

Sedation _____

What else helps? _____

Elimination

Bowels: Continent/Incontinent

How often opened? _____

Any medication? _____

Urinary: Continent/Incontinent

If incontinent: Day/Night/If not taken, how frequently? _____

Nocturia/Dysuria/Frequency/Urgency

Remarks _____ *Currently doubly incontinent* ____

Female patients — Menstruation

Post-menopausal   Taking the pill

Regular   Irregular

Amenorrhoea   Dysmenorrhoea

Next period due: _____

Uses: STs Tampons

Hearing

Hearing aid: YES/NO

Remarks _____

Vision

Glasses/~~Contact lens~~: YES/~~NO~~

Remarks _____ *For reading* _____

Oral

Dentures or crowns: YES/~~NO~~

Any problems with mouth or teeth?

_____

Mobility

Help needed with:

Walking/Standing/In/Out of bed/Bathing/Dressing/

In/Out of chair

Feeding/Other: _____

Remarks _____ *Unconscious - so totally* _____
_____ *dependent*

Prosthesis/appliance

Type of appliance _____

Help needed _____

General appearance

Normal	Dehydrated	Acutely ill
<u>Obese</u>	Thin	Emaciated

Remarks _____

Skin

<u>Satisfactory</u>	Broken areas	Dehydrated
Rash	Oedematous	Jaundiced
Pallor	Other _____	
	(including bruising)	

Remarks _____

Level of consciousness

Orientated   Semi-conscious

Confused   <u>Unconscious</u>

Remarks _____

Mental assessment (if appropriate)

Mood

Elated	Irritable	Agitated
Cheerful	Anxious	Aggressive
Miserable	Withdrawn	Suspicious
Apathetic		

Thought content

Hallucinations/Delusions/Paranoid Ideas

_____

Orientation

Time/Place/Person

Very confused   Slightly confused

Any particular time of day? _____

Confabulation _____

Remarks _____

Surveillance   Physical/Emotional

Information obtained from _____ *Mrs Anne Revons* ____

Relationship to patient _____ *Warden of flat.* _____

By _____

Position/level of training _____

Date _____ *06·02·87* _____

Time _____ *14.30* _____

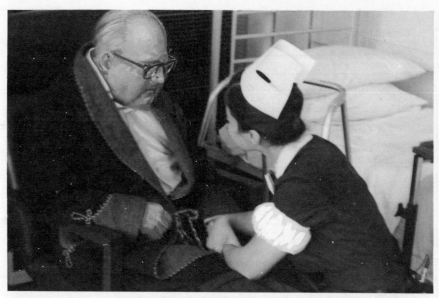

When taking a nursing history it is most important that the nurse explain the reason for the interview to the elderly patient so that he is aware that the information he gives will be purposefully utilised in planning his care. Often the elderly are not used to being interviewed, to being asked very personal questions, to explaining their anxieties or their problems; unless adequate explanation is given, they may be suspicious of the nurse's intentions in seeking such information. Once a good rapport has been established with a patient, however, much useful information may be gained more informally and naturally from conversations during general nursing procedures such as bathing or dressing practice. The nurse working with the elderly needs to develop the skill of open-ended questioning to allow her patients to elaborate upon their answers; thus information not anticipated but useful nonetheless may be obtained. Material that may be seen as extraneous in other settings is useful from the elderly patient — it may give clues to his emotional status, it may indicate his grasp of reality and priorities. A further skill the nurse has therefore to develop is the art of listening: not only to what is said, but how it is said: not only to what information is volunteered, but what is withheld. She must be alert to non-verbal clues a patient may give in terms of facial expression, posture and gesture.

With elderly patients with sensory loss the nurse needs to employ her full range of skills to overcome communication difficulties. She should ensure that the deaf patient has his hearing aid in position, tuned to the correct setting; she should sit in front of him and speak slowly and clearly at face level to facilitate lip reading. The blind or partially sighted patient may be dependent upon more frequent verbal responses or physical touch as he is deprived of seeing the facial expression or gesture that implies acceptance of his answers and encourages further speech. For patients with speech problems, time and patience are essential and a paper and pen to hand may be useful for the patient who can write responses. With all elderly patients, but especially with those with a communication problem, it is worth persevering when trying to obtain a nursing history — even if gaps have subsequently to be filled in with information from elsewhere. It implies that, accepting his disabilities, the nurse is interested in and concerned for him, and can form the basis of a trusting relationship.

The use of appropriate language is most important when interviewing elderly patients. 'What drugs do you take?' may produce the rather shocked response 'Oh, none at all', whereas 'Do you have to take tablets or medicines for anything?' may reveal a number of the former prescribed by the GP and one or two of the latter bought over the counter. Discussion of elimination may be difficult for some of the elderly, especially if there is any degree of incontinence present. Questions should avoid the censorious impression of 'Are you incontinent at all?'; a sympathetic enquiry about any difficulty experienced if the patient is not able to get to the lavatory easily is much more acceptable and will generally encourage fuller discussion of the situation.

To gain a comprehensive impression of the elderly patient, in her nursing history the nurse has seven areas of interest; they may be represented diagrammatically as in Figure 11.2.

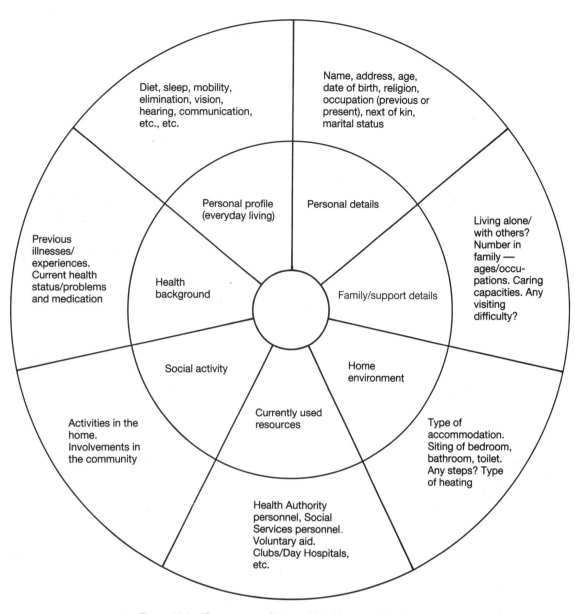

Figure 11.2 'Seven areas of interest' in taking a nursing history

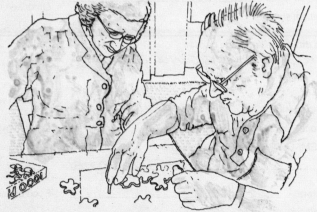

PAUSE FOR THOUGHT

The nursing history shown in Example 2 (Table 11.2) was taken on the admission to hospital of 86-year-old Mr Albert James and illustrates these seven areas of interest.

While the reason for obtaining personal details is perhaps obvious, taking the other six areas in turn, of what importance are they for the overall assessment of the patient and thus for the planning of care?

Table 11.2   Example 2

NURSING HISTORY AND ASSESSMENT SHEET
Record No. _039724_

PATIENT LABEL
Mr/~~Mrs/Miss~~ _Albert James_
Address _Flat 2 Brook House_
Braydon Road
Bristol

Male/~~Female~~   Age _86_
Date of Birth _10·03·01_

Date of admission/first visit
_06·04·87_
Time _11·25_
Type: ☐ <u>Routine</u>   ☐ Emergency
Transfer from: _____

Religion _Baptist_
Practising/baptised _Yes_
Minister _Rev. H. Small_
Telephone number _Bristol 695201_

Next of kin (name) _Alice James_
Relationship to patient _Daughter_
Address _As above_

Telephone numbers _Bristol 694372_
Contact at night/in emergency   YES/NO

Occupation (or father) _Retired Shopkeeper_
Marital status _Widower_
Children (or place in family) _Daughter + 1son in_
America
Other dependants _—_
Pets _Cat_
School (children only) _—_
Hobbies _—_
Clubs _—_
Favourite pastime _Watching television_

Does patient smoke?   YES/<u>NO</u>

Speech difficulty/language barrier
Speech rather indistinct at times.

Dysphasia   Dysarthria

Accommodation _With daughter for 4 years_
Lives alone   YES/<u>NO</u>
Part III/EMI/Old People's Home/Rented
Other _Flat (2 bedrooms)_

Consultant _Dr. Lloyd_
House officer _Dr. Smith_
Presenting condition _Parkinsonism_
Recurrent falls

History of present complaint and reason for admission
Treated for Parkinsonism for 2 years
Several falls in last month. Daughter (64)
recently had hip replacement - cannot
cope. Admitted after domiciliary visit
by Dr Lloyd/Staff Nurse Taylor

Past medical history
Myocardial infarction 1970. Small
stroke (left side) 1978. Parkinsonism
2 years.

Allergies _Penicillin_

Current medication
Madopar 250 daily

What patient says is the reason for admission and attitude to admission
"Been falling a lot - Alice not well"
Patient's expectations _"Get right and go home"_
Any problems at home while/because patient is in hospital?

Relevant home conditions (e.g. stairs)
Ground floor flat - one step at front door
Commode at bedside. Gas central heating
Visiting problems
Daughter staying with cousin until
17·04·87 (contact on Newport 779034)

Care at home
Community nurse _Sister Faunham_
No. _Bristol 629733_
Name of GP _Dr Payne_
Address _Patchway Surgery_
Other services involved
Home help _× 3 weekly_   Day hospital _× 2 weekly_
Laundry _____   Day centre/club _____
Inco supplies _____   Health visitor _____
Aids _____   Social worker _Church_
Meals on wheels _____   Voluntary worker ✓

Daily living

Diet
Special _—_
Food or drink dislikes _Dislikes cheese and_
tomatoes
Appetite: ☑ GOOD   ☐ POOR
Remarks _Used to main meal in evening_

Sleep

How many hours normally? _9-10_

Sedation _Sleeps well - settles at_

What else helps? _about 22.00_

Elimination

Bowels: Continent/Incontinent

How often opened? _3-4 x weekly_

Any medication? _"opening medicine"_
usually   _occasionally_

Urinary: Continent/Incontinent

If incontinent: Day/Night/If not taken, how frequently? _____

Nocturia/Dysuria/Frequency/Urgency

Remarks _Needs to pass urine two hourly_
v. occasionally incontinent at night.

Female patients — Menstruation

Post-menopausal   Taking the pill

Regular   Irregular

Amenorrhoea   Dysmenorrhoea

Next period due: _____

Uses: STs Tampons

Hearing

Hearing aid: YES/NO

Remarks _Deaf in right ear -? due to_
wax impaction

Vision

Glasses/Contact lens: YES/NO

Remarks _Two pairs - reading and distance_

Oral

Dentures or crowns: YES/NO

Any problems with mouth or teeth?
Top set only

Mobility

Help needed with:

Walking/Standing/In/Out of bed/Bathing/Dressing/

In/Out of chair

Feeding/Other: _____

Remarks _Can eat unaided if food cut up_

Prosthesis/appliance

Type of appliance _Walking stick_

Help needed _____

General appearance

Normal   Dehydrated   Acutely ill

Obese   Thin   Emaciated

Remarks _Some tremor observed at rest_

Skin

Satisfactory   Broken areas   Dehydrated

Rash   Oedematous   Jaundiced

Pallor   Other _Bruising - right arm_
(including bruising) _and buttock_

Remarks _2cm. red/broken area - right heel_

Level of consciousness

Orientated   Semi-conscious

Confused   Unconscious

Remarks _____

Mental assessment (if appropriate)

Mood

Elated   Irritable   Agitated

Cheerful   Anxious   Aggressive

Miserable   Withdrawn   Suspicious

Apathetic

Thought content

Hallucinations/Delusions/Paranoid Ideas
_____

Orientation

Time/Place/Person _Orientated_

Very confused   Slightly confused

Any particular time of day? _____

Confabulation _____

Remarks _____

Surveillance   Physical/Emotional

Information obtained from _Patient, Miss James,_
Medical notes.

Relationship to patient _Daughter._

By _____

Position/level of training _____

Date _06.04.87_

Time _12.15_

(a) Family/support details

It is important to investigate the family situation in order to assess:

1. The support previously received.
2. That currently available if home care is planned.
3. That available on discharge after hospitalisation.

As personal health problems or other commitments may preclude supporting an elderly relative, the nurse must ascertain not only which family members are living at home or in the near vicinity but also their ages and caring capacities. Information on the somewhat delicate area of family relationships

— unless volunteered by the patient or relative — is best gathered by observation rather than direct questioning.

A further consideration is that questioning may reveal a patient's anxieties — perhaps about potential problems where home care is planned ('I'm worried about the effect on Martha, she's not very strong, you know') or about a situation left at home if admission has been necessary (such as a disabled spouse being left alone). Visiting problems with a direct bearing on the hospitalised patient's emotional well-being may also be discovered. Possible concern regarding a pet should not be underestimated; not infrequently the elderly depend heavily on the companionship of dog, cat or budgie and anxiety about the care of the animal may considerably affect progress — sometimes to the extent of the patient refusing admission to hospital if satisfactory arrangements for care cannot be made.

In Example 2, Miss James had cared for her father for the four years since his wife's death, However, she had recently undergone major surgery herself and she could not cope satisfactorily when his condition deteriorated. There were no other relatives at hand to help, her only brother living and working in America, and it was decided to admit Mr James for a period of intensive rehabilitation. While he was in hospital she was going to stay with her cousin in South Wales for a short holiday; it was hoped that her father's condition would improve sufficiently for them to resume their previous living situation after her return.

(b) Home environment

Where home care is planned, an assessment must be made as to how conducive the environment is for home nursing; where hospitalisation is required, information on the situation from which the patient has come and to which he will return is equally important.

When a comprehensive idea of the environment has been obtained, three questions need to be asked.

1. Does it in any way contribute to the patient's problem or disability? For example: Is it damp or cold, increasing the risk of hypothermia? Is the toilet inaccessible, with resultant incontinence? Are safety hazards, such as paraffin stoves, putting the patient at risk?
2. What adaptations, if any, have been made to accommodate the patient's disability? For example, is there a commode at the bedside?
3. What further adaptations would assist with care or increase independence? (For example, moving a bed downstairs; provision of a ramp at the front door.)

For Mr James and his daughter the suitability of the environment had had to be considered from both their points of view; in addition to his problems, prior to her hip replacement, his daughter had been seriously disabled by osteoarthritis and they had been rehoused by the local authority in a two-bedroom, ground-floor, centrally heated flat. As Mr James could not reach the lavatory unaided, the community nurse had obtained a commode for him for bedside use at night.

(c) Currently used resources

An idea of the degree of dependency experienced before illness or admission to hospital can be gained by investigating the resources utilised in the community. Where home care is planned, it may be necessary to increase some sorts of provision — perhaps the home care assistant coming in on four days a week instead of two. In cases of hospitalisation, although facilities may be temporarily unused, links can be maintained with the different agencies to ensure continuity of provision when they are again required.

If valuable time and effort are not to be wasted, it is most important that agencies involved in an elderly patient's care be aware of all changes in circumstance; thus the ward sister on Mr James's admission cancelled his ambulance transport for his twice weekly Day Hospital visits and asked Miss James to let the Home Care Assistants Organiser know of his admission and her plans for a short holiday.

(d) Social activity

It is obviously important to know of the patient's areas of interest in order to maintain these if at all possible during illness or hospitalisation; a knowledge of his social activities is also useful, however, in judging how far frailty or disability permits him to socialise and participate in his local community. Although he had apparently been a very outgoing person in earlier years, Mr James's condition had increasingly isolated him and at the time of admission he was confined to the flat other than on his twice weekly visits to the Day Hospital. Most of his time at home was spent watching the television.

(e) Health background

Relevant previous illnesses and hospitalisations need to be discussed — but these rarely extend back to the septic toe or measles suffered in childhood! Rather than the physical aspects of earlier problems — which will be primarily the doctor's concern — it is the patient's reaction to previous experiences and expectations consequent upon them that interest the nurse. Elderly patients may have been hospitalised following injury or for surgery many years ago; anxieties may be engendered by memories of situations long since past — restricted visiting, perhaps, or inadequate post-operative pain control. Such concerns need to be identified and dealt with reassuringly.

The effect of current health problems on both the patient and his family needs to be investigated and their knowledge of, and attitude to, disorders discussed; how realistic their fears or expectations are can then be evaluated. Although he was anxious on admission to hospital, Mr James was quite aware of the need for his admission and the objectives of the proposed treatment (*see* quotations on the nursing history sheet).

The patient's understanding of any drug therapy should be discussed and the names and dosages of medications recorded where possible. Mr James's daughter had brought with her her father's Madopar but did not know the name of the 'opening medicine' resorted to occasionally to promote defaecation; further discussion with his community nurse revealed that it was Dorbanex Syrup.

(f) Personal profile

As with all other age groups, a personal profile is essential if care is to be planned to approximate as closely as possible to the patient's usual daily routine and if potential problems are to be identified and acted upon. For many elderly, adherence to everyday living styles is especially important and where mental functioning is precarious it may mean the difference between coping and confusion.

Where a patient is admitted to hospital, some units utilise 'questionnaires' to assess mental status; the patient is asked a series of questions designed to test short- and long-term memory and orientation in terms of time, place and person. However, some doubts have been expressed as to the value of such questioning; the appropriateness of responses to queries put when taking a nursing history generally may be a better indication of personal competence than knowing the name of the current incumbent of 10 Downing Street!

Physical observations made when taking a nursing history will include base-line recordings of temperature, pulse, respiratory rate and blood pressure and a sample of urine will be obtained for analysis to exclude any abnormalities. The condition of the skin must be carefully examined and a check made on the state of nails, hair and mouth. Any problem noted requires specific description on the nursing assessment sheet; the site of any bruising, for example, and the size as well as the location of any broken areas of skin.

While the patient's appraisal of his mobility and self-care capacities is obviously important, they should also be objectively assessed, if his condition permits, when the nursing history is taken. Mobility assessment should include the ability to rise from bed, chair and toilet and to walk alone or with suitable aids. Efficiency in washing and dressing to an acceptable standard and independent eating are capacities checked during appropriate activities.

Planning care

The information contained within the nursing history and the observations recorded form the basis from which actual and potential problems are identified, goals set and intervention planned. This part of the process should be a joint exercise involving the patient and, if appropriate, his family, as well as the nursing staff. The encouragement of his active participation signifies respect

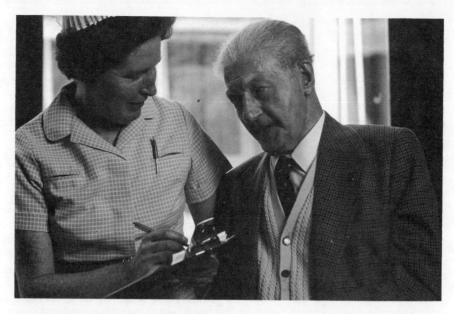

for his right as an individual to determine as far as possible his own health care and avoids any possible conflicts of interest. His smoking of 40 cigarettes a day, for example, may not be viewed by the elderly patient as a problem and the nurse, accepting this as his informed decision, should not make any attempt to persuade him to desist. This is not to dismiss the role of the nurse as a health educator: it is essential that patients be made aware of the injurious effects of behaviour such as smoking. But if the nurse recognises the elderly person as an autonomous individual, she must accept and respect personal decisions made. In a hospital ward, however, any possible risk to other patients because of a fire hazard is obviously the nurse's concern; the situation must be discussed with the patient and a compromise reached on where in the ward and under what circumstances his smoking is acceptable.

Urgent problems will receive priority and, as indicated earlier in the chapter, intervention may be necessary before a complete assessment has been made, decisions being taken on the basis of the patient's observable physical condition (e.g. correct positioning to maintain a patent airway in the unconscious patient). Existing problems and potential problems are then listed.

For each problem identified a goal will be set and a target date for its achievement indicated. It is vital that goals set be realistic in view of the patient's current capabilities and reasonably projected capabilities if over-optimism with consequent demoralisation is not to be engendered. Goals realisable in the short term (which can then be built on to reach longer-term ones) are more efficient motivators in the elderly when progress may be slow. Thorough assessment is an essential prerequisite as intervention must take into account all the variables; for the most part, elderly patients have multiple problems and any one may directly or indirectly affect the intervention planned to deal with any other.

An example here may serve to demonstrate the need to consider all aspects of a patient's problem:

> Eighty-four-year-old Mrs Adams had not had her bowels open for four days. On examination she was found to have a rectum loaded with hard faeces. A junior nurse assisting with her care was asked to suggest appropriate steps on the care plan for her patient and she put forward the plan given in Table 11.3.

Table 11.3   Care plan for Mrs Adams

Problem	Goal	Intervention	Evaluation
Patient has not had bowels open for 4 days	Short-term: Enable patient to have effective bowel action within 24 hours	Give two glycerin suppositories Give retention enema followed by evacuant	Very poor result Excellent result
	Long-term: Prevent constipation recurring	Encourage mobility Increase fluid intake Give high fibre diet	

As can be seen from the plan, the nurse correctly identified the problem, suggested a short-term goal and indicated the intervention to achieve this. This was implemented and Mrs Adams had an effective bowel action.

The nurse was then asked to look again at her long-term goal and the intervention indicated. While she could justify the inclusion of these nursing actions in general terms for preventing constipation (fibre adding bulk to the stool, etc.), for her specific patient she had overlooked three factors:

1. Mrs Adams was nursed on traction and therefore had very limited mobility.
2. Mrs Adams had severe congestive cardiac failure and therefore was permitted only restricted fluids.
3. Mrs Adams was edentulous and therefore had difficulty with fruit and vegetables.

In view of these factors the nurse's long-term goal was hardly a realistic one! Since her circumstances so predisposed Mrs Adams to constipation a more appropriate goal would have been to ensure that she had a bowel action at least every other day with the aid of suppositories if necessary.

For effective evaluation to be possible, the problems identified must be precise and the goals set and intervention planned must be specific and, where possible, measurable. For example, the frequently used phrase 'push fluids' is in itself meaningless; for the patient who is inadequately hydrated, however, the goal of an intake of not less than 2 litres daily, achieved by giving 150 ml of oral fluids hourly between 08.00 and 20.00 and 100 ml of soup before main meals determines very clearly what is to be done and how often, and permits objective evaluation of its effectiveness.

The purposes of a care plan have been defined[2] as:

1. Communicating information about the person/family and appropriate nursing actions and approaches.
2. Providing individualised and comprehensive care.
3. Providing coordination and continuity of care.
4. Facilitating ongoing and accurate evaluation of care.

An essential feature of the care plan if it is to fulfil these purposes is its ready accessibility for all involved personnel including the patient and his family. Where a patient is cared for in the community, the 'nursing notes' are left in the home and are thus also available to the GP, social worker and relief nursing staff; in hospital care the plan may be sited at the bedside or in a folder at the nurse's station.

Implementation

The intervention planned to achieve the stated goals may come into one of three categories; it may involve:

1. Doing tasks for the patient when he is unable to do them himself (phase 1 type care).
2. Helping the patient with activities where he is partially able to assist (phase 2 type care).
3. Strengthening the patient's own capacities where independence is possible (phase 3 type care).

Ongoing assessment is necessary to ensure that phase 2 type care is instituted as soon as the patient recovers some self-care capacity and he is not frustrated or lulled into a state of dependency because phase 1 type care is still given. The same applies as he progresses to phase 3 and complete independence. For example, bathing a patient may be a necessity in the early stages following a stroke when he is completely dependent; as soon as he is capable of assisting in the process, however, he is encouraged to do as much as he is able. Where a further degree of recovery occurs intervention may consist of the provision of

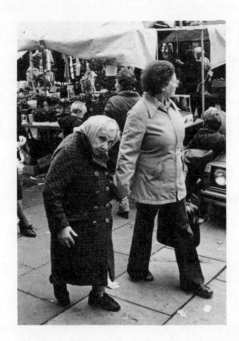

safety aids to enable him to bath unattended (i.e. strengthening his own capabilities). Equally important, of course, is the reversal of the process where a patient's condition deteriorates and increasing rather than decreasing levels of outside intervention become necessary.

It must be remembered that others as well as nurses are responsible for the implementation of care — often relatives or friends and the patient himself. They may require initial teaching, supervision and encouragement in this (*see* Chapter 10). Indeed, in the community a relative or friend may be the prime implementer of care, with the visiting nurse playing a supportive and guiding role. Where this is so, alternative approaches suggested by the other implementer as a result of experience or experimentation should not be regarded as threats but should be positively encouraged if to the benefit of the patient.

Evaluation

As the process of individualised care is a dynamic one, ongoing review of progress is essential, with care plans being adapted accordingly as the patient's situation changes. Just as he and his family should be involved in the planning and the implementation of care, their participation in evaluation should be encouraged. The focus of interest is on the problems which are resolving as well as those proving resistant to intervention and new ones arising as time goes by.

Where there is a satisfactory outcome to a problem, the intervention through which the goal was achieved should be discussed to ensure that it was acceptable to the patient and did not itself generate further difficulty. Walking the patient to the toilet two-hourly may have proved effective in preventing urinary incontinence but if the effort involved exhausted him and thus prevented him from joining in other activities, obviously a compromise would have been more acceptable with urinals offered two-hourly and a daily or twice daily walk to the toilet.

For problems which remain unresolved, the situation is reappraised to check that the basic need was initially correctly identified; when this has been ascertained, any new factors which could be exacerbating the situation are considered (has the onset of incontinence, for example, potentiated pressure sore development?). An honest appraisal of the quality of the prescribed care given must then be made; the optimum level may not have been possible for a variety of reasons and a reorganisation of staff or resources may be required to achieve it.

References

1. Collins, S. and Parker, E., *The Essentials of Nursing: An Introduction*, Macmillan Education, 2nd edn, 1987
2. Bower, F., *The Process of Planning Nursing Care: A Theoretical Model*, Mosby, 1972

Further reading

Pearson, A. and Vaughan, B., *Nursing Models for Practice*, Heinemann, 1986

Aggleton, P. and Chalmers, H., *Nursing Models and the Nursing Process*, Macmillan, 1986

Orem, D.E., *Nursing — Concepts of Practice*, McGraw-Hill, 1985

Henderson, V., *The Nature of Nursing*, Collier Macmillan, 1966

Roper, N., Logan, W. and Tierney, A., *Learning to Use the Process of Nursing*, Churchill Livingstone, 1981

Roper, N., Logan, W. and Tierney, A., *The Elements of Nursing*, Churchill Livingstone, 1980

A Systematic Approach to Nursing Care — An Introduction, Open University, Milton Keynes, Ref. **P553,** 1984

Chapter 12 Illness in the elderly

This text is not intended to cover in any detail the multiple pathological conditions from which the elderly may suffer; for comprehensive information on the disorders which affect this age group, the reader is referred to references 1 and 2. Suffice it to say here that, unlike their younger counterparts, elderly patients frequently show signs of several disease processes rather than one — some may be old, some new, some may be active, others inactive. And, again unlike younger patients, the elderly may show atypical presentations of disorders, with accurate diagnosis therefore requiring very careful investigation of very general symptoms.

The three 'Giants of Geriatrics' — conditions which bring about most breakdowns in family support and admission to hospital or residential care — have been defined as:

1. Intellectual failure.
2. Instability and immobility.
3. Incontinence.

These are not medical diagnoses in their own right but are symptoms of underlying disorders which, if promptly and correctly identified, are often amenable to treatment; they are used as a framework around which the remainder of this chapter is written, in close conjunction with Virginia Henderson's *Fourteen Components of Basic Nursing Care*.

PAUSE FOR THOUGHT

Recall the fourteen components of basic nursing care; consider those needs most likely to be experienced by elderly patients with intellectual failure, instability, immobility and incontinence.

The components of basic nursing care

These are the needs which the nurse attempts to meet regardless of the diagnosis. They involve helping the patient:

1. With respiration.
2. With eating and drinking.
3. With elimination.
4. To maintain the desirable posture in walking, lying and standing, and to help him move from one position to another.
5. With rest and sleep.
6. With the selection of clothing, and with dressing and undressing.
7. To maintain body temperature within the normal range.
8. To keep the body clean and to protect the integument.
9. To avoid the dangers in the environment, and to protect others from any potential dangers from the patient, such as infection or violence.
10. To communicate with others — to express his needs and feelings.
11. To practise his religion or to conform to his concepts of right and wrong.
12. With work or productive occupation.
13. With recreational activities.
14. To learn.

(after Virginia Henderson, 1960)

Obviously needs, being highly individual, will depend upon the particular patient and the degree to which he is incapacitated. The patient with mild intellectual failure, for example, may retain the ability to care for his own physical well-being largely independently; in the final phase of dementia, however, he will be totally dependent in every respect. The patient suffering instability because of joint pain may need help with movement; with rest and sleep; with hygiene, safety and socialising needs. However, if completely immobilised (perhaps after a fall), total dependency may again result. In addition to assistance with actual elimination and skin hygiene, and with dressing and undressing, the incontinent patient may require assistance because of the other factors which precipitate incontinence in the first place (such as instability, dietary inadequacies) and with resocialisation where the embarrassment of anxiety associated with the problem limited outside contact.

Intellectual failure

It is vital at the outset of the discussion of this problem to differentiate between acute confusional states and the progressive condition of dementia or chronic brain failure; the former are reversible with the appropriate treatment of the underlying factors, of which there are many. Confusional states are extremely common in the ill elderly and they have been described as being almost as non-specific as vomiting in a child.

Dementia, in which there is usually progressive impairment of the intellect and personality with resultant inability to care for physical and social needs, follows from pathological processes affecting the cerebral cortex. It will not be considered here in any detail as the unfortunate patient is generally cared for and his family supported by the psychiatrist and the psychiatric nursing team; the reader is referred to reference 3 for a full discussion of the multiple problems encountered.

Acute confusional states, as the term implies, are usually abrupt in onset with a previously coping, orientated elderly patient suddenly confusing people and events, places and times; the nurse may be mistaken for his long-dead sister and the ward be seen as the air raid shelter to which everyone must immediately go. The condition is often accompanied by restlessness and sometimes aggression if compliance from others is not obtained. Alternatively the patient may become withdrawn and anxious, deluded about events and surroundings; the elderly woman may become suspicious of her long-time neighbours coming in to help her or she may refuse admission to the doctor because he has brought imaginary 'other people' with him. In either type of situation there may be brief lucid intervals.

Confusion affects not only the patient: it can have a devastating effect on relatives or friends who may be at a complete loss to understand what is happening to a much loved and usually loving person. Not to be recognised, to be reviled with phrases never before heard from the patient, perhaps to be physically assaulted by her can shatter them and may precipitate aggressive behaviour in them, often directed at the staff rather than at the patient. In the hospital situation, confusion can also be disturbing and distressing to other patients and indeed to members of staff who are not used to dealing with it.

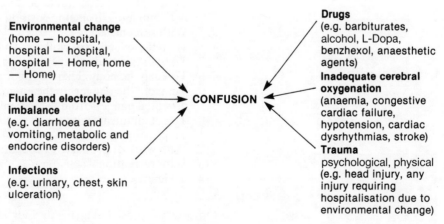

Figure 12.1   The confusing causes of confusion

The causes of confusion are so many and so varied they may well be described as the confusing causes of confusion! Rational explanations can be given where decreased cerebral oxygenation (perhaps due to anaemia or hypotension) results in confusion; the link between faecal impaction and disorientation, however, is less easily explained! Almost any physical or emotional stress can trigger off the problem in an elderly, unwell patient; the commoner causes are demonstrated diagrammatically in Figure 12.1.

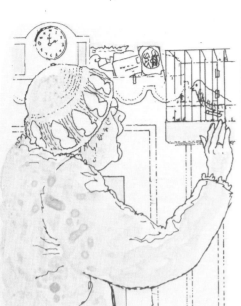

PAUSE FOR THOUGHT

Seventy-eight-year-old Mrs Davies lives with her son and daughter-in-law, having a bedsitting room on the ground floor of their house. Until a year before her admission she had been active in the local Senior Citizens' Centre and helped a lot in the house, her daughter-in-law being in full-time employment. Although maintaining her outside contacts since, in herself she had not seemed so well and her GP was treating her for mild congestive cardiac failure; her family put it down to her 'getting on'. Six or seven weeks before admission, however, it was obvious that she was becoming progressively more unwell and 10 days before she came into hospital she began to be confused especially at night, getting up at 02.00 to make breakfast and clean out the budgie's cage. A blood test — taken with some difficulty as she had become very hostile towards the GP — revealed that she was anaemic and she was admitted for investigation and treatment.

From the information on the nursing history and assessment sheet in Table 12.1, can you identify Mrs Davies's problems on admission and design a care plan for her?

Table 12.1   Example 1

NURSING HISTORY AND ASSESSMENT SHEET
Record No. _____065321_____

PATIENT LABEL

~~Mr~~/Mrs/~~Miss~~ _Ellen Davies_

Address _1 Blackdown Avenue_
Stoke Lodge
Bristol

Male/**Female**   Age _78_

Date of Birth _06.04.09_

Date of admission/first visit
_07.04.87_

Time _11.00_

Type: ☑Routine ☐Emergency

Transfer from: _____

Religion _Church of England_

Practising/baptised _Not Practising_

Minister _____/_____

Telephone number _____/_____

Next of kin (name) _John Davies_

Relationship to patient _Son_

Address _As above_

_____

Telephone numbers _Bristol 354673_

Contact at night/in emergency YES/~~NO~~

Occupation (or father) _Retired Housewife_

Marital status _Widow_

Children (or place in family) _1 Son 1 Daughter_

Other dependants _____/_____

Pets _Budgie_

School (children only) _____/_____

Hobbies _Knitting_

Clubs _Over 60's Club twice weekly_

Favourite pastime _Knitting_

Does patient smoke? ~~YES~~/NO

Speech difficulty/language barrier
None

Dysphasia   Dysarthria

Accommodation

Lives alone ~~YES~~/NO

Part III/EMI/Old People's Home/Rented
Lives with son and daughter-in-law

Consultant _Dr Lloyd_

House officer _Dr Smith_

Presenting condition _Anaemia_
Congestive Cardiac failure

History of present complaint and reason for admission

Unwell six weeks. Off her food.
Breathless on exertion, tired "no energy"
Confused at night for past week
Admitted at G.P's request.

Past medical history

Partial gastrectomy at age 60
Mild congestive cardiac failure for
twelve months.

Allergies   *None*

Current medication

Digoxin 125 slow-K Frusemide 40mg
2 tabs daily

What patient says is the reason for admission and attitude to admission

Tearfull – "I'm not well"

Patient's expectations   *"I want to go home"*

Any problems at home while/because patient is in hospital?

Relevant home conditions (e.g. stairs)

Has bedsitting room on ground floor
of house. Bathroom upstairs. Commode at
night
Visiting problems *Son and daughter-in-law both*
working - can visit evenings only

Care at home

Community nurse _____

No. _____

Name of GP   *Dr. Humphrey*

Address   *Stoke Lodge Health Centre*

Other services involved

Home help _____	Day hospital _____
Laundry _____	Day centre/club *weekly 2x*
Inco supplies _____	Health visitor _____
Aids _____	Social worker _____
Meals on wheels _____	Voluntary worker _____

Daily living

Diet

Special _____

Food or drink dislikes *Dislikes spicy food.*
Usually enjoys cheese, fish, milk.

Appetite: ☐ GOOD ☑ POOR

Remarks *Daughter-in-law has been giving*
sherry before meals.

Sleep

How many hours normally? *6-7 (Recently only 3-4)*

Sedation _____

What else helps? *Milky drink*

Elimination

Bowels: Continent/~~Incontinent~~

How often opened? *Every other day*

Any medication? _____

Urinary: Continent/~~Incontinent~~

If incontinent: Day/Night/If not taken, how frequently? _____
Passes urine 2-3 hourly

Nocturia/Dysuria/Frequency/Urgency

Remarks *Up to pass urine twice nightly*

Female patients — Menstruation

Post-menopausal	~~Taking the pill~~
~~Regular~~	~~Irregular~~
~~Amenorrhoea~~	~~Dysmenorrhoea~~
~~Next period due.~~	
~~Uses: STs Tampons~~	

Hearing

Hearing aid: ~~YES~~/NO

Remarks *Hearing good*

Vision

Glasses/~~Contact lens~~.   YES/~~NO~~

Remarks *For reading/television (2 pairs)*

Oral

Dentures ~~or crowns~~:   YES/~~NO~~

Any problems with mouth or teeth?

Sore tongue, mouth cracked at corners

Mobility

Help needed with:

Walking/~~Standing~~/~~In/Out of bed~~/Bathing/~~Dressing~~/

In/Out of chair/

~~Feeding~~/Other: _____

Remarks *Breathless on exertion needs to take time*

Prosthesis/appliance

Type of appliance   *None*

Help needed _____

General appearance

~~Normal~~	~~Dehydrated~~	~~Acutely ill~~
~~Obese~~	Thin	~~Emaciated~~

Remarks _____

Skin

Satisfactory	~~Broken areas~~	~~Dehydrated~~
~~Rash~~	Oedematous	~~Jaundiced~~
Pallor		
	Other _____	
	(including bruising)	

Remarks *Swollen ankles. Pressure areas intact*

<table>
<tr><td colspan="2">

Level of consciousness

~~Orientated~~   ~~Semi-conscious~~

Confused   ~~Unconscious~~

Remarks _See below_

Mental assessment (if appropriate)

Mood

~~Elated~~   ~~Irritable~~   ~~Agitated~~

~~Cheerful~~   Anxious   ~~Aggressive~~

~~Miserable~~   ~~Withdrawn~~   Suspicious

~~Apathetic~~

Thought content

Hallucinations/Delusions/Paranoid Ideas

Thinks G.P. "wants done with me"

</td><td>

Orientation

Time/Place/Person _Cannot give day/date or location._
knows personal details,
~~Very confused~~   Slightly confused _family members etc._

Any particular time of day? _Night time_

Confabulation _____

Remarks _____

Surveillance   Physical/Emotional

Information obtained from _Patient + Mrs Jean Davies_

Relationship to patient _Daughter-in-law *_

By _____

Position/level of training _____

Date _07·04·87_

Time _12·00_

*NB Relatives are extremely anxious about patients condition.

</td></tr>
</table>

Table 12.2 shows part of the care plan which was drawn up and put into practice following Mrs Davies's admission.

Table 12.2   Care plan for Mrs Davies

Problem	Goal	Nursing intervention	Rationale
1. Patient is confused, especially at night	Patient will feel comfortable and unthreatened in ward environment	One nurse to care for patient over span of duty	New faces compound confusion
		Explain all procedures, stay with patient and reassure during tests	Reduces anxiety
		Remind patient of location and purpose of hospitalisation	Assists with orientation, reduces anxiety
		Dress in own clothes, ask relatives to bring in personal effects from home	Reinforces self-identity. Retains link with home
		Adhere as closely as possible to normal daily routine	Continuity with usual lifestyle prevents further confusion
		At night — give milky drink to settle with (23.00)	Usual routine
		DO NOT REQUEST PRESCRIPTION OF NIGHT SEDATION	Sedation frequently exacerbates confusion
		Leave shaded light at bedside	Darkness in unfamiliar environment confusing
		Assist to commode at bedside as required	Usual routine
2. Relatives very anxious	Relatives will be able to discuss anxiety freely	Explain probable nature of confusion and objectives of care	Understanding lessens anxiety
		Make appointment to see house officer as soon as possible	Permits full explanation of medical problem, investigations, treatment
		Involve as much as possible in patient's care	Promotes sense of usefulness/ involvement (also for patient, continuity of care)
3. Mobility restricted because of breathlessness	Patient will mobilise without discomfort	Allow plenty of time for all activities	
		Nurse in end bed next to bathroom/toilet	All points minimise necessary energy expenditure
		Use Ambulift for bathing	
		Ensure armchair right height/ depth for patient's use	
		Leave all requirements at hand	

Table 12.2 Continued

Problem	Goal	Nursing intervention	Rationale
4. Sore mouth gives pain on eating	Patient will remain free of oral infection and be able to eat comfortably	Give two-hourly oral hygiene Encourage fluid intake (record on fluid balance chart), 1500 ml daily Apply prescribed cream to lips four-hourly	Removes sordes/freshens mouth Prevents cracking/entry of micro-organisms
5. Dietary intake less than 1000 calories in 24 hours	Patient will eat three meals daily totalling 1500 calories	Encourage patient to choose diet from menu Order small portions of desired foods Request prescription of glass of sherry before meals Present food attractively at table Give milk-based beverages as desired	Promotes interest in meals Larger portions off-putting Alcohol is an appetite stimulant
6. Discomfort from pitting oedema of ankles (28 cm)	Ankle swelling will reduce by 4 cm	Elevate feet on footstool when in sitting position Give prescribed diuretics as directed	Gravitation assists reduction Increases fluid output

Problems 1 and 2 were regarded as priority ones as they were causing such distress to the patient and her relatives. Over the first few days Mrs Davies's mental state fluctuated, with periods of lucidity interspersed with episodes of confusion; they continued to occur mainly at night. They were managed by talking reassuringly to her, bringing her to the nurse's station for a drink, ensuring that she emptied her bladder and then helping her back to bed. On the one occasion when she refused to return to bed, she was made comfortable in an armchair in the Day Room and eventually fell asleep there. Although remaining anxious about her, her son and daughter-in-law understood that in all probability the confusion was a transient feature of a treatable condition and they obviously benefited from the unbroken nights of sleep they were able to resume following her admission.

The results of a Schilling test and a bone marrow puncture indicated that Mrs Davies was suffering from pernicious (Addisonian) anaemia and treatment was begun with Neo-Cytamen (hydroxocobalamin). As her general condition improved she was able to join in diversional therapy activities, and although at first her concentration was poor, she began to quite enjoy these and within a week was not confused at all during the day. Ten days after treatment was begun, although still only sleeping spasmodically, she was also quite rational at night.

Unfortunately, the day after admission Mrs Davies developed oral thrush *(Candida albicans)*, which made her even less willing to eat. She was given chlorhexidine mouthwashes after meals and the infection was treated with nystatin suspension and lozenges; disposable crockery and cutlery were employed to prevent the spread of the infection. There was a corresponding improvement in both her oral and her general condition, however, and by the time of her discharge she was again enjoying small meals.

As her anaemia improved with treatment, the signs and symptoms of her congestive cardiac failure resolved and within three weeks she was largely self-caring and anxious to go home. Her family were delighted with her progress and also anxious for her discharge. Arrangements were made for medical follow-up by her GP (whom she then described as 'such a nice man!'), with the community nurse calling monthly to give the Neo-Cytamen injections which she will require for the rest of her life.

Instability and immobility

(a) Instability

'Once you're going, you've got to go' — a remark frequently heard from the unstable elderly. Because of defective balance and righting mechanisms, once they begin to fall they are unable to regain their previous posture. Unless this instability in the elderly is adequately dealt with, immobility may well ensue either because of fear of falling or because the trauma of an actual fall confines

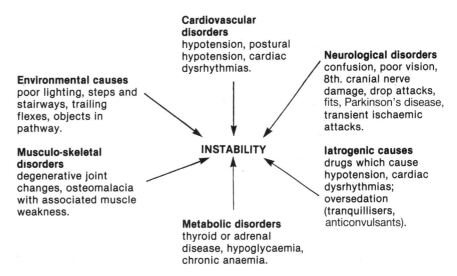

Figure 12.2 The causes of instability

the patient to bed or chair. Thus the causes of instability and their treatment demand some consideration here. As with confusion, they are multiple and often a combination of factors is involved (e.g. poor eyesight combined with inadequate lighting on a steep staircase) (*see* Figure 12.2).

1 Complications of instability

Confidence and mobility often ebb rapidly with the onset of falling. Stability may be sought in the home by holding on to furniture — a source of danger in itself if it is pulled over on top of the elderly person as he falls. Venturing outside the home may cease entirely with all the concomitant practical and social problems.

The injuries sustained in a fall may be of a major or a minor nature in general terms; however, for the elderly person the discomfort from even minor injuries such as bruising may be sufficient to take him to his bed with a rapid decline into immobility. Often such patients are seen in Accident and Emergency Departments following the fall but are discharged as 'no bony injury' is discovered. It is essential that appropriate analgesia be given and definite, prompt follow-up arranged.

Major accidents may result in multiple factures or severe burns if a stove or a fire is involved. Where the patient, although relatively unhurt by the fall, is unable to rise from the floor again and is forced to remain immobile until found by neighbours or other callers, hypothermia and pressure sore formation become real dangers, with possibly disastrous outcomes.

2 A patient study

Although too big for her and in a poor state of repair, eighty-two-year-old Miss Freda Webster would not leave the Victorian house in which she had been born and bred. For some time, her increasing frailty had been a cause of some concern to the few relatives she had left but she remained defiantly independent, refusing — politely but definitely — all offers of assistance from the community health and social services staff.

As she got out of bed one night to visit the lavatory, Miss Webster fell and was unable to rise again from the floor. She lay there until her nephew called on his way home from work the following evening; anxious because he received no reply and because the curtains were closed, he broke in through a window and found her. She was wearing only a vest and nightdress and was semi-conscious and very cold. Her GP was called and her admission to hospital was arranged immediately.

On admission Miss Webster was still semi-conscious and she was vomiting intermittently. Her rectal temperature was 31.2°C. Her priority needs were assessed and care put into practice as shown in Table 12.3.

When her temperature had risen to 33.5°C, Miss Webster was noticed to be twitching and runs of ventricular ectopic beats were observed on the oscilloscope. A blood test detected hypoglycaemia (which often occurs as the temperature of a hypothermic patient rises) and intravenous dextrose was given

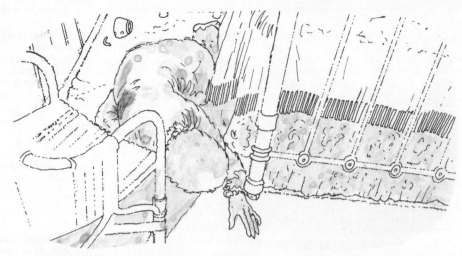

with good effect. An infusion of saline was commenced to keep the line patent in case further drugs should be necessary; a careful check was kept to ensure that it was absorbing only slowly and not overloading the circulation.

Twenty-four hours after her admission Miss Webster was alert and able to tolerate warm fluids by mouth with no further vomiting. The oxygen therapy, intravenous infusion and cardiac monitoring were discontinued; her rectal temperature was 35.5°C and vital signs were observed two-hourly for a further 12 hours. She was able to ask for bedpans as required.

Three days after admission her condition was greatly improved and she was sitting out of bed eating and drinking normally. She was badly bruised down

Table 12.3   Care plan for Miss Webster

Problem	Goal	Nursing intervention	Rationale
1. Patient hypothermic (rectal temperature 31.2°C)	Body temperature will rise by 0.5°C hourly to 36°C	Nurse in side ward with fan heater to bring room temperature to 25°C Wrap in blanket underneath bedclothes Check and record temperature half-hourly — rectal lead in position to electric thermometer	Slow rewarming essential to prevent vasodilation with further fall in blood pressure Rectal temperature most accurately reflects core temperature. Electric thermometer use saves disturbing/exposing patient unnecessarily
2. Vomiting with danger of aspiration	Patient will not aspirate vomitus	Nurse flat in semi-prone position Suction to hand — apply gently as required	
3. Respirations shallow and irregular (8/min) — potential problem of chest infection	Patient's respirations will increase to 14/min and chest will remain clear	Give oxygen via face mask at 4 litres/min Administer prophylactic antibiotics as prescribed	Endotracheal intubation avoided if at all possible — danger of ventricular fibrillation
4. Potential cardiovascular complications: (a) cardiac dysrhythmias (b) hypotension	Prompt recognition of problems allowing remedial action	Observe cardiac rhythm on oscilloscope — report dysrhythmias immediately Check and record pulse rate and blood pressure half-hourly Maintain vein patency with slow infusion as prescribed for any required therapy	Dysrhythmias commonest cause of death in hypothermia If blood pressure falls, rewarming may have to be slowed down
5. Unable to alter own position in bed: (a) reddened area on sacrum (b) potential pressure sore formation elsewhere	(a) Skin integrity will be maintained (b) Pressure areas will remain intact and unreddened	(a) Do not allow to lie supine Keep area as dry as possible Observe carefully (b) Turn two-hourly from side to side	Relieves/alternates site of pressure
6. Incontinence of urine due to semi-conscious state	(a) Patient will remain dry and comfortable (b) Patient will not lose further body heat in wet bed	(a) Nurse on absorbent incontinence sheets — observe half-hourly and change if wet. Apply barrier cream (b) DO NOT WASH EXTENSIVELY until temperature has risen	Prevents skin maceration Washing encourages heat loss

her right side, on which she had fallen, and analgesics were given regularly to relieve her discomfort. On beginning to mobilise her, however, it was apparent that her confidence was badly shaken; she became very agitated and refused to walk at all unless two nurses or physiotherapists were supporting her. She became tearful if a discussion of the problem was attempted.

Distressed by this tremendous change in Miss Webster, her great-niece determined to find the root of the problem and eventually persuaded her to discuss her fears. She was desperate to retain her independence but terrified of repeating her experience; she recalled with great clarity the early hours of her sojourn on the bedroom floor before she became semi-conscious — she had been sure she was going to die there. She was afraid that she would not be allowed home again anyway if her walking was seen to be so unstable and that she would 'be put away in a home'.

The great-niece was invited to the weekly ward case conference at which Miss Webster's progress was discussed. The physiotherapist, believing that she could become mobile again, felt there was some degree of urgency to motivate her to become so if further problems were not to arise. The medical social worker agreed to talk to her about the possibility of sheltered accommodation in a warden-controlled flat. At first Miss Webster flatly refused even to consider such a proposition but two days later she agreed to go with the social worker to look at one. On her return to the ward, she was obviously impressed with what she had seen and anxious to work on her mobility. Intensive physiotherapy was commenced and within a fortnight Miss Webster was ambulant with the aid of a Zimmer frame; she was taught how to get up unaided in the event of a fall. A flatlet fortunately became available in a block of sheltered accommodation only a short distance from her nephew and his family and she was able to move in straight from the hospital three weeks later.

In conclusion, the management of instability can be summarised under three headings:

1. The provision of a safe environment with ready access to assistance if required.
2. The recognition and adequate treatment of medical conditions predisposing to instability.
3. The provision, where appropriate, of stability aids (Zimmer frames, walking sticks, tripods).

Since 90% of falls in the home affect old people and since some 95% of accidents in geriatric units are due to falls, in sheer numerical terms their importance is obvious. In terms of the anxiety and the suffering they impose, however, they are worthy of even greater consideration.

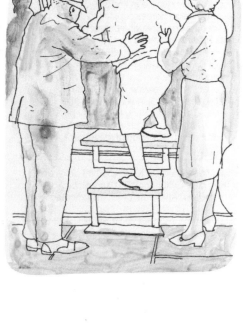

(b) Immobility

'Going off her feet', as the early phase of immobility is often described, is a common presenting feature of illness in the elderly and — as with intellectual failure and instability — there are many possible underlying causes (Figure 12.3). Urgent investigation and the institution of appropriate treatment is required as the complications of the condition often rapidly set in and make rehabilitation a more difficult proposition.

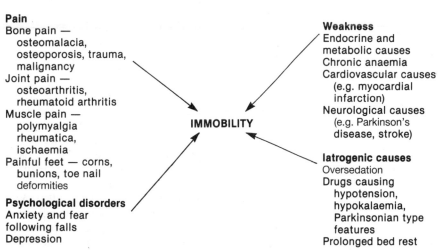

Pain
Bone pain — osteomalacia, osteoporosis, trauma, malignancy
Joint pain — osteoarthritis, rheumatoid arthritis
Muscle pain — polymyalgia rheumatica, ischaemia
Painful feet — corns, bunions, toe nail deformities

Psychological disorders
Anxiety and fear following falls
Depression

IMMOBILITY

Weakness
Endocrine and metabolic causes
Chronic anaemia
Cardiovascular causes (e.g. myocardial infarction)
Neurological causes (e.g. Parkinson's disease, stroke)

Iatrogenic causes
Oversedation
Drugs causing hypotension, hypokalaemia, Parkinsonian type features
Prolonged bed rest

Figure 12.3   The causes of immobility

Table 12.4   The complications of immobility

Complication	Cause	Nursing intervention
Pressure sores	Prolonged pressure with tissues compressed between bone and firm surfaces Friction damaging skin Incontinence leading to maceration	Identification of at-risk patients (*see* Scoring Chart, Table 12.5). Regular and frequent alteration of position. Keeping skin clean and dry. Correct lifting to prevent shearing forces causing friction. Careful bedmaking. Ensuring balanced diet to promote healthy tissues
Contractures	Owing to disuse, muscles shorten by fibrosis and joint fixations occur	All joints put through full range of movements at least three times daily — passive exercises if patient unable to cooperate, active if he is. Application of splints as indicated (must be individually made, well fitting to prevent pressure sores). Warmth and analgesia with gradual extension if painful limitation of movement occurring
Constipation/incontinence	Inactivity leads to reduced appetite and slowing of gut motility. Accumulating faecal mass may cause urinary incontinence/spurious diarrhoea (see following section)	Encourage fluid intake, at least 1500 ml daily, and high fibre diet. Ensure comfort and privacy for toilet purposes. Aperients given as indicated
Thrombo-embolism	Venous stasis leading to deep vein thrombosis and possibly pulmonary embolism	Avoid dehydration by encouraging fluid intake as above. Limb movements at least three times daily — passively or actively

Infection
  Urinary
 	
  Chest
	
	Urinary stasis (inadequately emptied bladder). Possibly secondary to incontinence
	Restricted respiratory movements. Difficulty in expectoration
		
		Encourage fluid intake. Regular vulval/penile toilet Privacy and comfort for toilet purposes
		Support adequately to permit full chest expansion. Assist with deep breathing/coughing exercises

Apathy and depression	Restricted physical and mental horizons	Diversional therapy. Provision of conducive company

Table 12.5 'Scoring Chart' for identifying patients at risk of developing pressure sores (devised by Norton et al., 1962)[4]

Physical condition		Mental condition		Activity		Mobility		Incontinence	
Good	4	Alert	4	Ambulant	4	Full	4	None	4
Fair	3	Apathetic	3	Walk/help	3	Slightly limited	3	Occasionally	3
Poor	2	Confused	2	Chairbound	2	Very limited	2	Usually/urine	2
Very bad	1	Stuporous	1	Bedfast	1	Immobile	1	Doubly	1

When a patient's condition is assessed on all five points, if his total score is 14 or below, he is considered 'at risk' of developing pressure sores. The tool should be used in ongoing assessment as, when a patient's condition deteriorates and he has a falling score, it is again indicative of an increasing risk.

In addition to preventing the complications of immobility, the nurse will be involved in investigations to ascertain the exact cause of the problem and in the treatment of this once it has been found. Treatment may be relatively simple — perhaps the organisation of thorough pedicure to deal with painful feet — or it may be very complex — perhaps a combination of drug therapy and radiotherapy to control bone pain from metastases; in either instance, the patient will require assistance with remobilisation and practice in the activities of everyday living once more.

Incontinence

(a) Urinary incontinence

Psychologically and sociologically the consequences of loss of continence in our society should never be underestimated. The loss of dignity and self-esteem precipitated by losing control and wetting bed, chair or clothing can have devastating effects upon the individual concerned. In the community many families attempt heroically to deal with incontinence and all that it entails but not infrequently its onset heralds the breakdown of a support system and the admission to hospital of the elderly person.

Physiologically, incontinence as an entity requires qualification as the term covers a wide spectrum of urinary problems, including the stress incontinence experienced on coughing or sneezing (perhaps due to uterine prolapse), the 'dribbling' incontinence an elderly man may have following prostatectomy and the urge incontinence occurring because the elderly person cannot reach the lavatory in time. Many incontinent patients can, with the correct treatment, regain their continence and, even where the condition proves irremediable, management to permit comfort, dignity and socialisation should be an achievable objective.

At this point, the reader may find it useful to review the physiology of micturition (covered in Pat Hunt and Bernice Sendell's book in the Essentials of Nursing course, entitled *Nursing the Adult with a Specific Physiological Disturbance*), and also the age-related aspects of excretion discussed in Chapter 2 of this book.

(b) The maintenance of continence

It is an unfortunate fact that many elderly patients continent on admission to hospital lose their continence in the days following admission. Prevention, as always, is better than cure and all steps must be taken with a newly arrived patient to promote the maintenance of continence.

> **PAUSE FOR THOUGHT**
>
> Why do you think that incontinence may become a problem on admission? What nursing intervention must be instituted to prevent it becoming so?

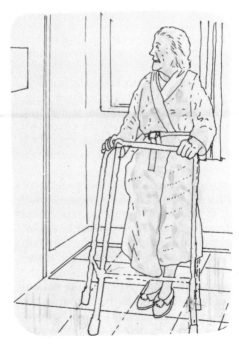

Reduced bladder capacity requires most elderly people to visit the lavatory fairly frequently; generally at home their environment is adapted for them to cope with this or their daily routine is planned to take account of it. In an unfamiliar environment, however, ready access to facilities may not be available and, where his condition confines him to bed or chair, the patient is dependent upon nursing assistance which he may be reluctant to request; alternatively he may not know how to do so. Drug therapy or the effects of the patient's illness itself may lessen consciousness of the need to micturate or the ability to do so in the right place at the right time.

If continence is to be maintained, on admission the nurse in taking her nursing history must ascertain the patient's normal bladder habits; the usual frequency of micturition both by day and night must be established and any difficulty with the activity noted. Any drug therapy likely to affect the patient in this respect is similarly noted. The patient's physical ability to use the available toilet facilities must be assessed and any anxieties identified. The nurse call system should be explained and demonstrated and assurance given that a call will be answered promptly.

Care can then be planned to take account of the patient's norms and capabilities with facilities offered at the usual times or when micturition is anticipated (e.g. after short-acting diuretics have been given). Special care of course must be taken with patients with communication difficulties (such as aphasia following stroke, or confusion) when interpretation of non-verbal signs such as restlessness or anxiety may be required; these are both frequently indicative of a patient's need to pass urine. One very practical consideration for the ambulant patient taking himself to the toilet in an unfamiliar environment is to permit easy recognition of the relevant rooms — in some units the toilet doors are painted a very distinctive bright colour to assist him!

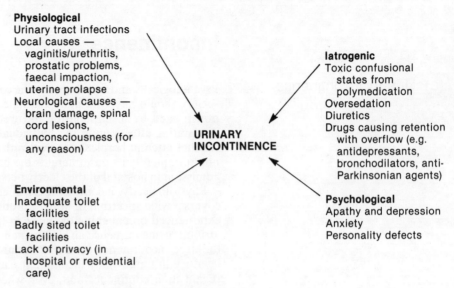

Physiological
Urinary tract infections
Local causes —
    vaginitis/urethritis,
    prostatic problems,
    faecal impaction,
    uterine prolapse
Neurological causes —
    brain damage, spinal
    cord lesions,
    unconsciousness (for
    any reason)

URINARY INCONTINENCE

Iatrogenic
Toxic confusional
    states from
    polymedication
Oversedation
Diuretics
Drugs causing retention
    with overflow (e.g.
    antidepressants,
    bronchodilators, anti-
    Parkinsonian agents)

Environmental
Inadequate toilet
    facilities
Badly sited toilet
    facilities
Lack of privacy (in
    hospital or residential
    care)

Psychological
Apathy and depression
Anxiety
Personality defects

Figure 12.4   The causes of urinary incontinence

(c) Investigation

Urinary incontinence in an elderly person at home or in hospital requires thorough investigation and appropriate treatment of the underlying cause wherever possible (Figure 12.4). Environmental difficulties will be considered and urine tested for glucose (a common cause of urethritis); a midstream specimen will be cultured to exclude infection. Vaginal examination in the elderly woman may indicate ageing changes which are mirrored on the (structurally similar) urethral epithelium and which respond well to hormone replacement therapy; it may also reveal uterine prolapse, with the displacement mechanically irritating the bladder. Rectal examination is required to exclude faecal impaction with the mass pressing forward on the bladder outflow; in the elderly man it may reveal prostatic enlargement. Where no local or infective cause can be found for the incontinence in the mentally alert elderly person, cystoscopy and cystometric studies may be carried out to check the competency of the bladder structures and control mechanisms.

(d) Management of urinary incontinence

As important as the practical skills of those caring for the incontinent patient are their attitudes to the problem. Regaining bladder control may be a protracted affair and a professionally sympathetic manner and determined optimism are essential. Only when these are present in the nurse can they be infused into the patient and his family.

Where a treatable cause is found for the patient's incontinence, medical management will be directed at correction of the underlying problem (e.g. surgery for uterine prolapse, antibiotics for infection, alteration in the drug regimen). Often as an ill elderly patient's general condition improves, his incontinence spontaneously clears. Habit retraining may still play an important part in rehabilitation, however, and may prove effective where incontinence persists despite medical treatment.

In habit retraining the aim is to discover the patient's own pattern of micturition and to reinforce it with the offer of toilet facilities as required until his regular habit of urination is re-formed. Various charts have been designed to record the patient's voiding pattern. Initially observation is made hourly of the patient's condition — continent or incontinent; in either event facilities are offered and it is noted if urine is passed (a refusal to use the facilities is also noted). Over the period of a few days, on close inspection of the chart the patient's pattern emerges. If, for example, on three days running the patient passes urine into the toilet at 10.00, this will continue to be a time when facilities are offered; if, on those three days, although dry at 11.00, the patient was found to have been incontinent by 12.00, facilities are obviously offered at 11.30 in an attempt to 'catch the patient'.

For some patients who fail to show any regular pattern of voiding, two-hourly toileting may impose an artificial habit to which the bladder may, over a period of time, adjust.

The expertise of other members of the multi-disciplinary team must also be utilised in the management of the incontinent patient. The prescription of drugs such as Cetiprin (emepronium bromide) which improve bladder capacity may be useful especially at night. The physiotherapist assists with the promotion of mobility, which may in itself overcome the problem; she also has a range of techniques for improving pelvic muscle control, which may prove especially beneficial with elderly women. The occupational therapist can provide appropriate aids to enable easier toileting and can advise on the adaptation of clothing to minimise delay in using facilities. It must be remembered that correct dress in itself is an incentive to the regaining of continence and the ambulant patient should always be appropriately clothed.

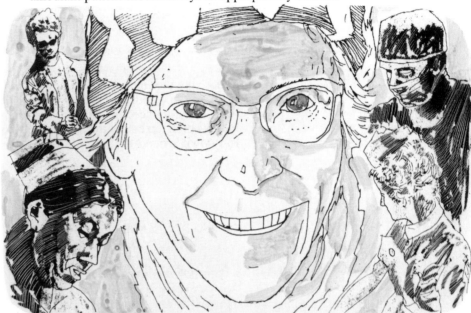

While habit retraining is being carried out or where incontinence continues to be a problem, the use of protective pads and pants to safeguard the patient's skin and dignity is indicated. A particularly efficient variety for both men and women are Kanga pants, with their waterproof marsupial pouch into which a doubled pad is inserted which absorbs the urine flow, leaving the actual fabric of the pants' gusset dry. The pads are changed (without removing the pants) and disposed of as necessary and the pants washed and dried as normal underwear. It is important that the correct size pants are used for each individual patient (as they must be close fitting) and that overfilling of the pad is not allowed to occur; thus the frequency of pad changing must be determined by experience. The pants can be successfully worn in bed, with the pad positioned a little further back in the pouch.

Appliances used where incontinence proves intractable include sheath devices for men and indwelling urinary catheters for both sexes; confusion, however, makes their use impractical. In view of infection risks, catheterisation is sometimes deprecated; where it will significantly improve the quality of a patient's life, however — perhaps allowing care at home where otherwise hospital care would be required — it is generally agreed that it is both acceptable and advisable. Not infrequently, incontinent patients deliberately restrict their fluid intake in the mistaken belief that this will reduce the problem; it may in fact exacerbate it by predisposing to constipation and urinary tract infections. An important aspect of nursing care is the encouragement of an adequate intake — at least a litre and a half daily. It is vital where a patient has an indwelling catheter in position if blockage is not to prove troublesome.

(e) Faecal incontinence

Incontinence of faeces is extremely distressing for the elderly patient and often very difficult for relatives to deal with in the community situation. The cause must be quickly sought and brought under control (Figure 12.5).

By far and away the most common cause of faecal incontinence in the elderly is constipation! Naturally this would appear to be a contradiction in terms; the

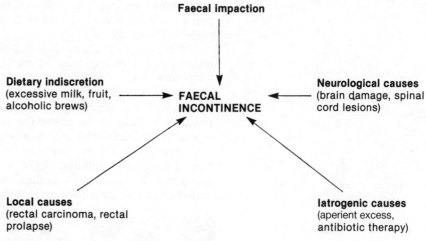

Faecal impaction

Dietary indiscretion
(excessive milk, fruit,
alcoholic brews) ──→ **FAECAL
INCONTINENCE** ←── Neurological causes
(brain damage, spinal
cord lesions)

Local causes
(rectal carcinoma, rectal
prolapse)

Iatrogenic causes
(aperient excess,
antibiotic therapy)

Figure 12.5   The causes of faecal incontinence

underlying mechanism is as follows. Prolonged periods with no bowel action result in the withdrawal of fluid from the faecal mass through the large bowel wall; the stool becomes progressively harder and more difficult to pass. The faeces at the top end of the impaction become liquefied by bacterial action and run down around the side of the mass to trickle uncontrollably through the anus.

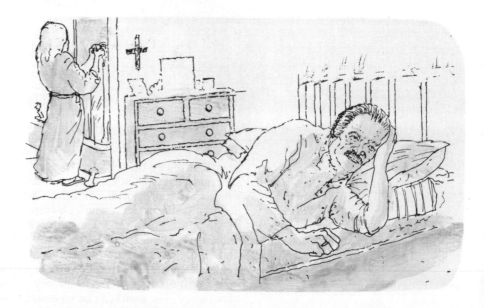

PAUSE FOR THOUGHT

85-year-old Mr Stephan Petovitch and his 84-year-old wife live in a very close-knit Polish community in the city centre. Their GP — who had had little previous contact with them — was called to see him when he had been confined to bed for a week with influenza; he found him doubly incontinent with obvious faecal impaction. On her initial visit the community nurse found Mr Petovitch depressed and tearful in bed, his wife overwrought and exhausted and piles of soiled sheets in the bath. Can you identify the priority needs of the patient and his wife in this situation?

Their needs could be summmarised as follows:

Patient's needs

1. Relief of lower bowel obstruction and prevention of recurrence.
2. Institution of regular toileting to regain bladder control.
3. Skin hygiene and relief of pressure to preserve integrity.
4. Remobilisation.

Wife's needs

1. Laundry service.
2. Provision of necessary equipment (commode, incontinence pads).
3. Assistance with physical care and household tasks.

Mr Petovitch's faecal impaction was dealt with by the administration of an olive oil retention enema followed by an evacuant; some faeces remained in the rectum at the end of the procedure and required manual removal by the nurse. The importance of preventing a recurrence was explained to both him and his wife and advice was given on fluids and diet. He was bed-bathed and comfortably positioned before the nurse left. She arranged for the provision of a laundry service and the delivery of a commode; a supply of pads was left in the house. Mrs Petovitch would not accept the services of a home care assistant but contact was made with the parish priest, who organised voluntary assistance for her.

Visits were made by one of the community nursing staff daily for a week to assist with toileting, skin care and remobilisation. The administration of glycerin suppositories to promote bowel action was initially necessary, but as Mr Petovitch's mobility improved and his dietary intake increased, a satisfactory bowel habit was established by use of the commode or toilet immediately after breakfast (utilising the gastro-colic reflex). Regular toileting virtually eliminated his urinary incontinence, with only the occasional 'accident' at night.

Visits were gradually decreased as Mr Petovitch's condition improved. A community auxiliary continues to visit fortnightly to assist with bathing, however, and the community sister visits monthly to monitor the situation.

References

1. Coni, N., Davison, W. and Webster, S., *Lecture Notes on Geriatrics,* Blackwell, 1980 [new edition now in preparation]
2. Hodkinson, H.M., *An Outline of Geriatrics,* Academic Press, 1981
3. Brooking, J.I., Dementia and confusion in the elderly. In Redfern, S. (editor), *Nursing Elderly People,* Churchill Livingstone, Chapter 18, 1986
4. Norton, D., McLaren, R. and Exton-Smith, A.N., *A Investigation of Geriatric Nursing Problems in Hospital,* National Corporation for the Care of Old People, 1962

Further reading

Mace, N.L. and Rabins, P.V. with Castleton, B.A., Cloke, C. and McEwan, E., *The 36-hour Day — Caring at Home for Confused Elderly People,* Hodder and Stoughton with Age Concern, 1985

Directory of Aids, 2nd edition, Association of Continence Advisors, London, 1984

Norton, C., *Nursing for Continence,* Beaconsfield Publishers, 1986

Chapter 13   Surgery and the elderly

Despite the multiple pathology from which they frequently suffer and their reduced tolerance of shock, many elderly patients respond remarkably to well planned surgical intervention with perceptive and skilled nursing support. Where operation offers a worth-while improvement in the quality of life for the patient — as may hip replacement for the elderly woman immobilised by osteo-arthritis — age in itself should be no barrier to its performance. It should certainly not be so when an otherwise fit elderly person has a condition which, if left untreated, may give rise to an emergency situation with all its concomitant problems at a later, perhaps less healthy, stage; the 69-year-old man will respond more favourably to the elective repair of his inguinal hernia now than to the emergency operation necessitated by its strangulation in six or seven years' time.

This having been said, however, it is equally important that where an elderly patient is already severely handicapped his wishes and those of his family should be sought before only dubiously beneficial or perhaps 'heroic' surgery is contemplated. Resection of colon and formation of colostomy may not be the appropriate treatment for an 86-year-old woman with dementia who is brought to the Accident and Emergency Department with intestinal obstruction, for example. It is vital that the totality of the patient's situation be appreciated — in terms of functional ability, mental status and social support — before clinical and nursing management decisions are made.

Assessment and pre-operative care

In order that a thorough check can be made on the patient's pre-operative condition, he should be admitted several days before elective surgery is planned; the time during which X-rays, electrocardiograms and blood tests are taken and drug therapy assessed and perhaps reviewed is also time for the elderly patient to acclimatise to the new situation in which he finds himself, the ward routine and its personnel. Post-operative confusion, not infrequently experienced by the elderly, is much lessened when the patient is familiar with his environment.

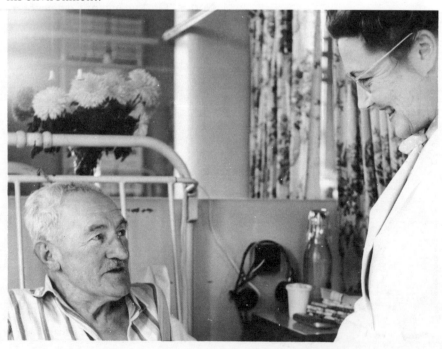

Careful — and often repeated — explanation of all procedures is vital, and apprehension must be recognised and allayed by discussion and appropriate intervention. There may be concern about a situation left at home — perhaps an elderly disabled spouse who cannot use public transport to visit — or about financial or other affairs not left in order. Liaising with other personnel to deal with such matters — the medical social worker in the first instance or the hospital administrator should the patient wish to make a will in the second — is an integral feature in pre-operative preparation.

When surgery is planned there is time to ensure that the patient is in the best possible condition pre-operatively; time, for example, to reduce obesity (which contributes greatly to the development of post-operative complications), to correct dehydration or to improve nutrition (and thereby to promote more ready wound healing). Where it is foreseen that the operation will leave the patient with an altered body-image, perhaps following mastectomy, amputation of a limb or creation of a stoma, it should be realised that the psychological trauma precipitated at any stage of life may well be compounded by the age factor and the appropriate specialist (appliance officer, stoma therapist) should see the elderly patient beforehand. An initial relationship in which any anxieties can be discussed can then be formed and post-operative care and support explained. A realistic but optimistic approach must be adopted by all involved in the patient's care; difficulties may well be inevitable but, if the patient is to be motivated to work at his recovery, they must be seen to be manageable, not insurmountable.

Attention is paid to all general pre-operative nursing measures such as identification of the patient, recording of base-line observations of temperature, pulse, respiratory rate and blood pressure, urine analysis, skin preparation and encouragement of exercises taught by the physiotherapist. Removal of aids and prostheses should not unnecessarily compromise the patient's dignity or independence — a hearing aid, for example, may be vital for adequate communication with an elderly deaf patient right up to induction of anaesthesia and it should not be removed before leaving the ward simply for 'convenience'. Similarly, co-operation will not be forthcoming post-operatively unless the aid is resited as soon as the patient regains consciousness! Starvation is less well tolerated by the elderly than by their younger counterparts, and excessive periods of giving nothing by mouth should be avoided; oral hygiene or frequent mouthwashes should be available to keep the patient comfortable while he is permitted nothing.

When toilet facilities have been offered and premedication has been given, the patient should be asked to remain at rest in bed as drowsiness may exacerbate frailty or unsteadiness. Depending on the type and the extent of the surgery to be performed, in some units prophylactic antibiotics and subcutaneous heparin are given to the elderly patient with his premedication to minimise the likelihood of the post-operative complications of chest and wound infections and deep vein thrombosis.

Emergency surgery

Emergency surgery precludes much of the above-mentioned preparation and the elderly patient may be bewildered and confused by his sudden illness or accident, rapid admission to hospital, subjection to urgent investigation and preparation for theatre. It is most important that the anxiety engendered by this situation in both the patient and his relatives should not be overlooked by staff preoccupied by his physical needs.

Both physiological and psychological complications are more likely to occur following emergency surgery; early recovery is potentially more hazardous and rehabilitation more prolonged.

Anaesthesia

While most surgery is carried out under a general anaesthetic, some operations may take place with other methods employed; certain types of ophthalmic surgery, for example, may be carried out under local anaesthetic and epidural anaesthesia may be used for older patients undergoing such procedures as

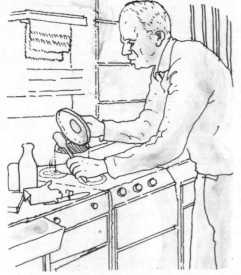

prostatectomy or hernia repair. For specific pre-operative preparation and post-operative care of patients receiving such treatment, the reader is referred to Reference 1.

PAUSE FOR THOUGHT

The following nursing history was taken from Mr Bruce Thomlinson on his emergency admission to hospital. He lives with his 75-year-old wife — who is severely incapacitated by arthritis — in a terraced house in an older part of the city; their children and their families live many miles away. In recent months the Thomlinsons have only used the ground floor of the house and they have had community support in the form of a home care assistant twice weekly and a community auxiliary fortnightly. Most of the shopping is done by a voluntary worker but Mr Thomlinson prepares all the meals.

Using the information given in Table 13.1, devise a pre-operative care plan for Mr Thomlinson, who is to undergo transurethral prostatectomy.

Table 13.1   Example 1

NURSING HISTORY AND ASSESSMENT SHEET

Record No. _043679_

PATIENT LABEL

Mr/~~Mrs~~/~~Miss~~ _Bruce Thomlinson_

Address _72 Austen Road_
St. Werburghs
Bristol

Male/~~Female~~   Age _78_

Date of Birth _11·05·05_

Date of admission/first visit
_16·05·87_

Time _15·45_

Type: ☐ Routine ☑ Emergency

Transfer from: _____

Religion _C/E_

Practising/baptised _Not practising_

Minister _/_

Telephone number _____

Next of kin (name) _Irene Thomlinson_

Relationship to patient _Wife_

Address _As above_

Telephone numbers _Neighbour - Mrs Hard 629043_

Contact at night/in emergency YES/~~NO~~

Occupation (or father) _Retired Docker_

Marital status _Married_

Children (or place in family) _3 (none live locally)_

Other dependants _—_

Pets _Dog_

School (children only) _—_

Hobbies _—_

Clubs _Wills Pensioners Association_

Favourite pastime _Reading_

Does patient smoke? YES/~~NO~~ _40 a day_

Speech difficulty/language barrier
None

Dysphasia   Dysarthria

Accommodation

Lives alone ~~YES~~/NO

Part III/EMI/Old People's Home/Rented

Other _Own House_

Consultant _Mr Horton_

House officer _Dr Reynolds_

Presenting condition _____
Acute retention of urine

History of present complaint and reason for admission
Dribbling urine, poor stream for several weeks
Unable to pass urine at all for 24 hours
Bladder distended, painful.
Admitted at G.P.'s request.

Past medical history
Inguinal hernia repair 1968
Myocardial infarction 1974
Chronic bronchitis - several years

Allergies _—_

Current medication
None prescribed

What patient says is the reason for admission and attitude to admission
"A blockage in the waterworks"

Patient's expectations _Operation - home as soon possible_

Any problems at home while/because patient is in hospital?
Wife has severe arthritis

Relevant home conditions (e.g. stairs)

Downstairs of house used only
Bathroom/toilet on ground floor.

Visiting problems _Wife cannot visit unless_
brought. Family not in Bristol.

Care at home

Community nurse _Sr. Jackson_

No. _367299_

Name of GP _Spiers_

Address _Charlotte Keel Health Centre_

Other services involved

Home help _x 2 weekly_	Day hospital _____
Laundry _____	Day centre/club _____
Inco supplies _____	Health visitor _____
Aids _____	Social worker _____
Meals on wheels _____	Voluntary worker _✓_

Daily living

Diet

Special _Soft diet - edentulous_

Food or drink dislikes _Does not like milk_

usually
Appetite: ☑GOOD ☐ POOR

Remarks _Has cut down fluid intake because_
of urinary problems

Sleep

How many hours normally? _6-7_

Sedation _None_

What else helps? _Guinness before bed_

Elimination

Bowels: Continent/Incontinent

How often opened? _Daily_

Any medication? _____

Urinary: Usually Continent/Incontinent

If incontinent: Day/Night/If not taken, how frequently? _____

Nocturia/Dysuria/Frequency/Urgency

Remarks _Self - retaining catheter in situ-_
inserted in A/E dept.

Female patients — Menstruation

Post-menopausal   Taking the pill

Regular   Irregular

Amenorrhoea   Dysmenorrhoea

Next period due:

Uses: STs Tampons

Hearing

Hearing aid: YES/NO _Left ear_

Remarks _Set on number 4_

Vision

Glasses/Contact lens: YES/NO

Remarks _2 pairs - distance and reading_

Oral

Dentures or crowns: YES/NO

Any problems with mouth or teeth? _Mouth dry_
Does not use his dentures

Mobility

Help needed with:

Walking/Standing/In/Out of bed/Bathing/Dressing/

In/Out of chair

Feeding/Other: _____

Remarks _Rather unsteady on his feet_

Prosthesis/appliance

Type of appliance _Uses walking stick_

Help needed _____

General appearance

Normal	Dehydrated	Acutely ill
Obese	Thin	Emaciated

Remarks _____

Skin

Satisfactory	Broken areas	Dehydrated
Rash	Oedematous	Jaundiced
Pallor	Other _____ (including bruising)	

Remarks _____

Level of consciousness

Orientated	Semi-conscious
Confused	Unconscious

Remarks _____

Mental assessment (if appropriate)

Mood

Elated	Irritable	Agitated
Cheerful	Anxious	Aggressive
Miserable	Withdrawn	Suspicious
Apathetic		

Thought content

Hallucinations/Delusions/Paranoid Ideas

Orientation

Time/Place/Person _Orientated_

Very confused   Slightly confused

Any particular time of day? _____

Confabulation _____

Remarks _____

Surveillance   Physical/Emotional

continued overleaf

The care plan given in Table 13.2 was that devised and used pre-operatively for Mr Thomlinson; yours should contain the same features. For post-operative care, see opposite.

Table 13.2   Care plan for Mr Thomlinson

Needs/problems	Goals	Intervention	Rationale
1. Anxiety re: (a) wife at home (b) admission to hospital (c) forthcoming treatment/operation	Will be able to discuss problems freely with staff without becoming unduly anxious	(a) Contact medical social worker (b) Introduce to patients, ward, etc. (c) Careful explanation of care, procedures, operation Allow time for questioning	Check mobilisation of community support Familiarity reduces anxiety
2. Difficulty with hearing	Will be able to communicate effectively with staff and others	Ensure hearing aid *in situ*, at correct setting Speak clearly at face level	Assists patient with lip reading
3. Safety in ward areas	Will be safe from dangers in the environment	Position bed at appropriate level Familiarise with ward layout Ensure walking stick to hand — check ferrule Keep patient area obstruction-free Request that patient smoke in Day Room only	Enables patient to transfer more safely Worn ferrule dangerous Prevents tripping Prevents fire hazard in bed/with oxygen therapy in ward
4. Dry mouth and reluctance to drink	Will drink at least 2 litres daily and not develop any oral infection	Give 150 ml fluid hourly — nature as desired Explain importance of increasing fluid intake Record intake on fluid balance chart Encourage mouthwashes after meals	Gain patient's co-operation
5. Patient is edentulous	Will be able to eat 3 meals daily	Assist with choice from menu of soft diet	
6. Thin build and limited mobility — danger of pressure sore formation	Pressure areas will remain intact and unreddened	2-hourly encourage mobility, alteration of position when in bed/chair Encourage fluid and dietary intake as planned above	To relieve/alternate sites of body pressure To maintain healthy tissues
7. Unable to bath unaided	Will manage hygiene needs as independently as possible	Use Ambulift for bathing Assist only as necessary Leave as desired	Preserve dignity and independence as much as possible
8. Self-retaining urinary catheter *in situ*	(a) Will feel no discomfort from catheter (b) Will not develop ascending infection	(a) Support tubing adequately (b) Maintain closed system Catheter care twice daily Encourage fluid intake as above	Dragging may cause pain from balloon at bladder outlet Prevent entry of pathogenic micro-organisms
9. Potential chest infection — heavy smoker, impending surgery	Chest will remain clear, no cough or pyrexia	Encourage reduction Encourage physiotherapy exercises, deep breathing/expectoration	
10. Patient is to undergo surgery	Will be prepared for operation	Ensure correct details identiband. Record base-line observations — temperature, pulse, respiratory rate, blood pressure Test urine and record result Give nothing orally six hours pre-operatively Shave operation site, bath, dress in operation gown, clean linen Give premedication as ordered Remove hearing aid after induction of anaesthesia	For post-operative comparison Exclude abnormalities Prevent aspiration of vomit under anaesthesia Reduce number of pathogenic organisms on skin Sedate patient, inhibit respiratory secretions Ensure effective communication until anaesthetised

Note: For further information on post-operative care, see Pat Hunt and Bernice Sendell's book in the Essentials of Nursing Course, entitled *Nursing the Adult with a Specific Physiological Disturbance.*

Post-operative management

Once consciousness has returned following anaesthesia, pain relief is important in order both to promote rest and to increase activity; the danger of over-sedation in the elderly is a real one, however, and regular but small doses of analgesics are prescribed. Morphine-based drugs and barbiturates are avoided, as the former may cause respiratory depression and the latter confusion in an older patient.

Vital signs must be carefully monitored and significant deviation from the patient's pre-operative norm should be promptly reported: even moderate hypotension is poorly tolerated by the elderly patient, who runs the risk of both cardiac and renal complications when this occurs. Intravenous fluids must be carefully regulated; circulatory overload easily happens and central venous pressure monitoring may therefore be employed. Fluid balance should be meticulously observed. Many elderly patients experience difficulties with elimination post-operatively — incontinence may be an early problem or retention of urine may necessitate the temporary insertion of a urethral catheter. Whenever possible, the patient will be more comfortable and be able to pass urine more easily if assisted out of bed to do so.

Early attention must be paid to measures to prevent chest infection, which may readily develop in an older patient with decreased chest expansion and a weaker cough reflex. As soon as his general condition allows he should be supported comfortably in the upright position and encouraged with his deep breathing exercises and expectoration; he should be shown how to give manual support to a chest or abdominal wound while doing so. Judicious timing of analgesia will make cooperation with the physiotherapist more realistic!

Intervention to maintain skin integrity is essential in the elderly patient who may have lain immobile on the operating table for some time. Alteration of position to distribute weight and thereby pressure is carried out hourly or two-hourly on return from theatre and accessories such as alternating pressure mattresses, bed-cradles and sheepskin pads or bootees may be employed. Correct lifting will obviate shearing forces damaging fragile ageing skin and ready attention to any incontinence or sweating will prevent maceration of sacral areas.

Early ambulation will assist in the preservation of skin integrity as well as lessening the risk of deep vein thrombosis and pulmonary embolism. However, it should be gentle and slowly progressive for the elderly patient, whose capabilities should not be overtaxed in the early post-operative period; fatigue may lead to frustration, loss of confidence and subsequent lowering of motivation. It is not encouraging dependency to assist as required in the activities of daily living at this time — support can be gradually withdrawn as the patient's ability to cope unaided returns.

Early introduction to any appliance or prosthesis is essential for the elderly patient. Although he may not be able to manage independently — for physical or emotional reasons — changing a colostomy bag or walking with an artificial limb, the psychological adjustment essential for successful rehabilitation can begin with its presentation. Thereafter, repeated explanation, reassurance and assistance with its management by nurse or therapist should encourage gradual acceptance and independence. If the patient himself is not able to become completely self-reliant, however, the help of a close family member may be enlisted or community nursing support arranged, as anxiety about potential problems on discharge will otherwise retard his progress towards it.

Reference

1. Shergold, L., Epidural and spinal anaesthetics, *Nursing Times*, **82,** No. 27, 2–8 July, 1986, 44–45

Further reading

Hunt, P. and Sendell, B., *Nursing the Adult with a Specific Physiological Disturbance*, Macmillan, 1987

Chapter 14   Drugs and the elderly

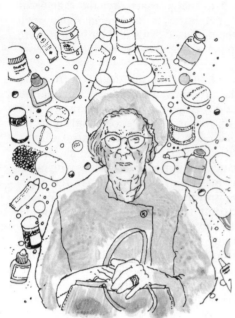

In a recent survey of the patients in one general practice,[1] 87% of the over-75-year-olds were receiving regular drug treatment and no less than 44% were taking three or more different drugs daily. This would appear to be reasonably characteristic of the elderly in the community as a whole and, when one considers the large number of drugs prescribed for hospital in-patients (an average of 4.6 drugs per patient in Scotland[2]), it is small wonder that a third of the NHS drug expenditure is invested in this age group!

Experiencing illness and disability more frequently than the younger members of the community and, in addition, suffering often from a multiplicity of health problems, the elderly may benefit greatly from selective and appropriate therapy. Occasionally, intervention may be life-saving — as with the administration of antibiotics in overwhelming infection — but more often it is directed towards enhancement of the quality of the patient's life. Thus the positive benefits to the patient of considered and well informed drug therapy should not be forgotten in the face of current concern regarding drug induced problems in the elderly; they may include independence as opposed to immobile dependency in the arthritic or physical and mental tranquillity as opposed to ongoing pain and consequent depression in the terminally ill.

Where problems do arise with drug therapy in older patients, there may be several contributory factors. These include the following:

(a) The altered presentation of disease in the elderly may mean that an incorrect diagnosis is acted upon.

(b) Pharmacokinetics (the time course of drug absorption, distribution and elimination from the body) and pharmacodynamics (the bodily response to drugs) are altered by the processes of ageing.

(c) Drugs given for one problem may exacerbate another in the patient with multiple disorders or the treatment of many separate problems may result in drug interaction.

(d) For a variety of reasons the patient may not take his drugs or he may not take them correctly.

The altered presentation of disease

A different reaction to illness is often seen in the ageing person, with a less florid and dramatic picture than that seen in a younger individual. It is sometimes said that in the elderly 'the organs suffer in silence': the patient may sustain a myocardial infarction but suffer no pain — only a transient giddiness; he may develop a chest infection but have no pyrexia — instead experiencing an acute confusional state. Accurate diagnosis is essential if inappropriate drug therapy is not to worsen the true condition.

Pharmacokinetics and pharmacodynamics

As has been discussed before, the elderly are not a homogeneous group in any way and there may be wide variation in tolerance of, and reaction to, drugs. However, in general, the following points should be kept in mind:

1. Absorption. Research has indicated that there is little appreciable change in the rate or the amount of drug absorption from the gastro-intestinal tract as a consequence of ageing. Where the ingestion of laxatives causes intestinal hurry, however, there may be inadequate absorption and a poor diet may retard the absorption of fat-soluble drugs.

2. Distribution. Changes in drug distribution within the body occur because of the reduction of total body water with ageing and the lessening of lean body mass with a corresponding increase in fatty tissue. Thus in the elderly there may be higher blood levels of water-soluble drugs and a longer duration of action of fat-soluble ones.
3. Elimination. Although a few drugs are excreted by the body in an unchanged form, most are reduced to less active or inactive metabolites by the liver; as liver function declines with ageing this process may be prolonged in older patients and nutritional deficiencies, smoking or substantial alcohol intake may further retard metabolism. Decreased glomerular filtration rate and tubular secretion slows down renal elimination. Many of the adverse drug reactions experienced by older patients (especially to Digoxin, beta-blocking agents and antibiotics) therefore follow from the prolonged higher tissue levels resulting from this belated elimination. Smaller dosages are generally prescribed in an attempt to overcome this difficulty.

Correspondingly fewer studies have been carried out in the area of pharmacodynamics, but ageing organs do appear to respond to similar drug dosages in a different manner from younger ones; in some cases the drug effect is decreased, in some potentiated. Certain drugs such as barbiturates, which the elderly are known to tolerate badly, are generally avoided.

Multiple pathology and multiple medication

When a patient requires treatment for several problems, the situation has to be assessed in its entirety, as medication given to deal with one condition may exacerbate another (e.g. phenylbutazone for arthritis may worsen heart failure or steroids may unmask latent diabetes) or multiple medication may lead to harmful drug interaction. The picture may be complicated by the patient, in addition to taking prescribed drugs, buying 'over the counter' medications of which the doctor is unaware; gastric sedatives, laxatives, analgesics and vitamins are often bought in large quantities by the elderly and all may interact with prescribed therapy.

The following brief case study illustrates some of the problems experienced by the elderly when multiple problems are treated with multiple medication:

> 72-year-old Mr Griffiths had been receiving clonazepam (Rivotril) and tetrabenazine (Nitoman) for three years to control arteriosclerotic chorea when he developed temporal arteritis and polymyalgia rheumatica. Large doses of steroids (prednisone) were prescribed but this treatment rapidly reactivated an old gastric ulcer and, on admission to hospital, metoclopramide (Maxolon) and cimetidine (Tagamet) were ordered to relieve his nausea and epigastric pain. When he became confused, developing faecal impaction and urinary incontinence, Dorbanex and emepronium bromide (Cetiprin) were added to his daily schedule.
>
> Over a period of a week Mr Griffiths's mental and physical condition deteriorated considerably but no physical cause for this could be demonstrated. The decision was made to discontinue all drug therapy with the exception of decreasing doses of prednisone.
>
> Within three days Mr Griffiths was fully alert, continent of urine and generally improving. Smaller doses of clonazepam and tetrabenazine were gradually reintroduced at a later stage when his chorea symptoms again became apparent.

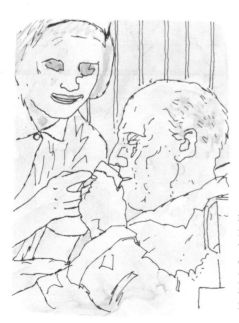

When the least possible number of drugs are given there will be correspondingly fewer errors in taking, adverse reactions and interactions. Patients receiving long-term medication require regular review — initially to ascertain whether continued therapy is necessary and, if it is, whether alteration in dosage is appropriate. When the chest infection which precipitated a patient's heart failure has satisfactorily resolved, for example, his Digoxin and diuretics may be discontinued; as the diabetic patient ages, his insulin requirement may well be less than in his younger years.

Correct drug-taking

In one survey of elderly patients discharged from hospital half were found to make errors in taking their prescribed medication in the first 10 days. Problems may arise:

1. When the drugs are not taken at all.
2. When an incorrect dose is taken.
3. When the drugs are not taken at the correct time.

PAUSE FOR THOUGHT

'Compliance' is the term used to indicate a patient's attentiveness to his doctor's orders with regard to drug-taking. What problems may an elderly patient experience which may result in difficulty with compliance?

For a variety of reasons the initial directions given concerning his medication may not have been fully understood by the patient. All too often, directions are given to the elderly in a busy GP's surgery or, in the ward, immediately prior to discharge; in the latter instance, the patient is frequently more concerned with gathering together his belongings, wondering about the transport arrangements made for him and anxious to get home. Any hearing impairment not taken into account will, in either situation, make the problem worse unless clear, unambiguous written directions, which the patient can read and refer back to later, are also given.

Errors in timing or dosage may follow from the patient with failing vision not being able to read the directions on the small labels affixed to drug containers. Forgetfulness may mean doses are omitted or sometimes duplicated, should the patient not recall having already taken his drugs. The 'childproof' containers which, in recent years, have contributed to the decrease in accidental poisonings at one end of the age scale have, however, resulted in some difficulties at the other, where arthritic hands may also find them 'granny-proof'! (Chemists can be requested to use other containers where this is known to be a problem.)

Certain presentations of drugs may not be acceptable to the elderly patient; large tablets may pose problems for those with swallowing difficulties and some powders are very unpalatable and may be omitted for that reason. Alternative presentations are often available (e.g. Dispersible Septrin in place of Septrin tablets) and may overcome non-compliance.

Sometimes difficulties are encountered because the elderly patient finds that prescribed medication adversely affects other problems which he has (e.g. taking diuretics exacerbates his urinary urgency and incontinence) and he discontinues his drugs of his own accord. As previously discussed, multiple problems require careful assessment and occasionally a compromise has to be reached between the patient and his doctor as to what treatment is necessary and what personal inconveniences or discomforts can be tolerated.

PAUSE FOR THOUGHT

Mrs Emma Burnside is a very independent 84-year-old widow who lives alone; she has been receiving treatment in the geriatric unit for congestive cardiac failure and varicose ulceration of the left leg. Despite restricted vision and a tendency to be rather forgetful, she is now largely self-caring and most anxious to return home.

What steps can be taken to try to ensure that her necessary medication will be taken following discharge?

For a week prior to discharge Mrs Burnside could be encouraged to care for and to deal with her own medication on the ward. While some staff could be strongly opposed to this, advancing many arguments concerning both practical and administrative difficulties in a ward situation, where trials have been carried out (for example, at the Royal Devon and Exeter Hospital) the fears of the staff were not realised; no patient took another's tablets, no major omissions occurred and the patients overall were found to benefit, proving far more competent on discharge.

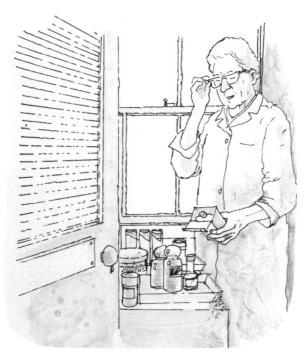

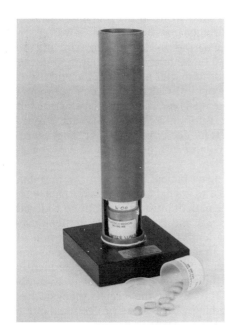

Fewer problems will occur if Mrs Burnside can take her medication in one daily dose. Specially large containers can be requested from the pharmacy so that larger labels can be affixed for more ready recognition, and colour coding of the bottles with a large corresponding chart to indicate the prescribed times of taking could help if more frequent doses are necessary. A page-a-day calendar, hung firstly by her locker and then by her tablets at home, from which she could tear off a page as a day's drugs were taken would help Mrs Burnside to avoid repetition of a dose.

Involvement of a willing neighbour or a nearby member of the family in her drug regimen — quite legitimately resorted to in some instances — may not be acceptable to Mrs Burnside with her independent nature. The two or three visits a week made by the community nurse to follow up the progress of her varicose ulcer, however, will provide the opportunity for unobtrusive monitoring of the situation. Should any problems be discovered, the situation can then be reassessed and an alternative plan formulated — perhaps utilising an aid such as the Lewisham Tablet Dispenser appropriately 'primed' by the nurse for the time between her visits. With this, the tablets are put into small plastic containers with the time marked clearly on the front. The containers are placed in the appropriate order in the cylindrical container and, as one dose is removed, the next one appears in view with the time at which it should be taken.

References

1. Law, R. and Chambers, C., Medicines and elderly people: a general practice survey, *British Medical Journal*, **i,** 1976, 565–568
2. Lawson, D. H. and Jick, H., Drug prescribing in hospitals: an international comparison, *American Journal of Public Health*, **66,** No. 7, 1976, 644–648

Further reading

Bleathman, C., Pharmacology, *Nursing*, **2,** No. 41, September, 1985 1213–1217

Medication for the elderly, *Journal of the Royal College of Physicians of London*, **18,** 1984, 7–17

Chapter 15   Dying and death

Contemplating the approaching death of his elderly father in 1952, Dylan Thomas wrote:

> 'Do not go gentle into that good night;
> Old age should burn and rave at close of day —
> Rage, rage against the dying of the light.'

Death as a subject, of course, is a popular one with poets; the sentiment expressed here, however, may be seen as one characteristic of an age group (Thomas was 38 when this poem was published) when facing up to the finite nature of human existence. Studies have shown that rarely are the elderly concerned about death itself, nor do they often consider it; that was a feature of earlier years when the end, with its apparent negation of a lifetime's work and effort, was at all costs to be denied. More frequently the well adjusted elderly have come to face the inevitable end of life with equanimity — but they do not anticipate it in any way which affects their living of the remainder of it.

Conscious awareness of one's own mortality may be aroused, however, by serious accident or illness or the death of a partner or close companion, and the need to discuss one's life and dying may then be felt; *dying* rather than *death*, since the manner of the end would appear to matter more than the end itself. There is a need in all of us to make sense of our living in the face of our dying; where achievements (small as well as great) can be recalled and satisfaction felt at a life well lived, contentment is the usual outcome. Only where wrongs remain unrighted and omissions regretted does bitterness or anger predominate. The integrity of old age (*see* Chapter 3), however achieved, eases the acceptance of one's mortality.

The nurse's responsibility towards the dying patient, at home or in hospital, is very great. There can be no second chance to amend errors in care, to make up for oversights; her care and support of the patient must be carefully considered to take account of his unique requirements and her plan then meticulously implemented. Her duty is no less to the patient's family, both during the time of his final illness and in their bereavement. In the days, months and indeed years to come the manner of a loved one's death and the care received are frequently recalled; there should be no cause for further sorrow or regret that all attempts were not made to achieve 'peace at last'. It is sad that the term 'euthanasia' has lost its original meaning, i.e. a good or a happy death; as a professional much concerned with the quality of living, the nurse must be equally concerned with the quality of dying.

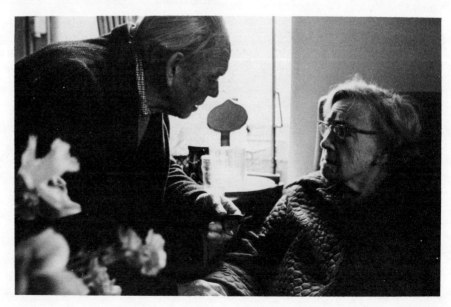

As in any other age group, death may come suddenly or may follow a short illness. For many elderly people, however, a prolonged period of dependency may precede the end of life. Thus the appropriate setting for care is an essential consideration. Against a tide of institutionalisation of important life events, a sweeping generalisation is sometimes made that 'home is the best place to die'; indeed for many it may well be but for others it may not be at all satisfactory and each person's individual circumstances, needs and desires must be carefully considered and discussed before decisions are made. Even then, since circumstances, needs and desires may change, contingency plans should be made should the elderly dying patient eventually require admission to hospital from home or should it be possible for a hospitalised patient to go home for his last few days if he and his family wish it.

Home care, where desired and possible, allows the elderly patient to remain in a familiar environment with the people who mean most to him, surrounded by the effects of a lifetime. Dying can be a lonely experience and the support of one's nearest and dearest is, as a rule, infinitely preferable to the company and ministrations of comparative strangers. That support, however, especially in a protracted final illness often with increasing immobility, incontinence and perhaps confusion, places great strain on the carer or carers. The principal carer may well be an equally elderly and less than healthy spouse; it may be a daughter or a daughter-in-law with considerable other commitments. Their physical, emotional and social needs cannot be forgotten; an appreciable degree of community support (from the Primary Health Care Team, Social Services department and voluntary bodies) must be available to them.

Admission to hospital in the early stages of the final illness may be necessary to confirm a diagnosis, to treat distressing symptoms or to establish a satisfactory management pattern (notably in terms of drug therapy) to facilitate home care. Later short-term admissions to allow the carer a week's or a fortnight's break may prevent long-term admission brought about by the exhaustion of her caring capacity. Where the elderly person is alone, however, or suitable conditions are lacking within the community, admission for ongoing hospital care is generally the appropriate decision and the nurse should spare no effort making the final home a peaceful and happy environment for the elderly patient.

For the dying patient the aims of nursing care are the alleviation of symptoms and the promotion of physical and mental comfort; for his family they are support — both practical and emotional — and protection from the hazards of bereavement. The degree of emotional support required should not be underestimated; often the extent of the physical caring commitment in the last stages of illness is appreciated but — because of the age of the dying person — the grief component may not be. Age is in this respect irrelevant; even when one is seventy and one's dying mother ninety, the child–mother bond is little changed from earlier years and the final separation can be equally devastating; after an intimate partnership of sixty years or more, the death of a spouse can effectively mean the end of one's own meaningful life as well. And anticipation of the event in no way lessens the shock of its actual occurrence. Assistance with 'grief work', before death with both the patient and the family, and after the event with those who remain, is an essential feature of the nurse's task.

The practical aspects of caring for the dying patient and his family are considered in *Essentials of Nursing: An Introduction* (Collins and Parker) of this series and at this point the reader is referred to the relevant section there. However, it is as well to reiterate that for each person the dying experience is absolutely unique and, while the nursing measures and medications to deal with pain, insomnia, anorexia, constipation, dyspnoea or any other symptom can be discussed in general terms, the overall totality of care for an individual and his family cannot. A dynamic care plan, adapted to meet the changing needs of all concerned, must, in its implementation, express to the patient: 'You matter because you are you; you matter to the last moment of your life and we will do all we can to help you not only to die peacefully but also to live until you die.'[1]

Bereavement

Rarely is grief first experienced at the moment of death; frequently it is encountered in a family in the days and weeks preceding the end when the inevitability is seen, the loss anticipated. Thus it is often shared with the dying person who is taking his leave of those around him. A tremendous mixture of emotions may be experienced by relatives — sadness, fear of being left alone, anger at the situation, with subsequent guilt, self-reproach for real or imagined failings in love or care — and thus a highly charged emotional atmosphere may exist in the home or hospital setting to which the caring team must be highly sensitive. Since suppression only serves to further weight the burden, expression of grief in any of its manifestations must be seen to be acceptable and encouraged appropriately.

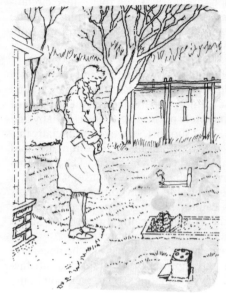

PAUSE FOR THOUGHT

Bereavement following a close relationship has been described as 'the most traumatic event in one's life — the cost of commitment'. What support may the bereaved person require (a) in the period immediately following death, and (b) in the weeks and months to come?

Again, individual needs must be assessed and appropriate response made, since differences in reaction to loss will be observed, these depending on many factors including emotional stability, previous experience of death and perhaps religious orientation. However, several common features are seen in grieving individuals of all backgrounds and the following paragraphs will be based on these.

Initial reactions to the death of a loved one include detachment (the situation being too painful to bear), numbness (all emotion drained away) and frenzied activity to keep oneself occupied. At this stage assistance with the practicalities associated with death must be available; in addition to 'not knowing what to do', the elderly bereaved may not physically be able to cope with the necessary tasks — obtaining medical certification of the cause of death, arranging for undertaker services, registration of the death and organisation of the funeral. When death has taken place in the home, the community nurse will assist with these practical aspects and liaise with the appropriate personnel. All too often, however, after the traditional cup of tea and organisation of transport home, hospital staff view their duty to the bereaved as discharged. Especially where an elderly person is returning home alone, contact should be made with the Primary Health Care Team so that immediate follow-up with any necessary help can be arranged.

The first phase of mourning usually involves concentration on the deceased and in the early days of bereavement there is often a great need to talk about the person, to relive times together — the good and the bad — and to go over and over the dying experience. Where community staff have been involved in care it is easier for them to offer support at this time — simply by their compassionate presence, their willingness to listen; contact made only following bereavement rarely permits such an effective relationship to be formed. Crying, anorexia, sleep disturbances and lack of concentration commonly occur; alternatively they may become more apparent after several weeks when the reality of the loss is more fully appreciated.

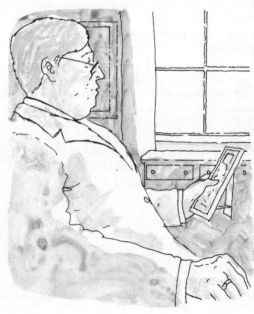

From centring on the deceased, the bereaved person's thoughts turn eventually inwards; there may be anger expressed towards the deceased or others and appeals for help in the despair that ensues. It is vital that the period of withdrawal and disorganisation — previously formalised in the mourning rituals of earlier generations — be respected and seen as normal if the person is to be able to work through his grief. A higher incidence of illness and death is seen in the first year following bereavement and the health, especially of the elderly mourner, should be closely monitored; evidence of apathy and self-neglect must be rapidly detected and steps taken to counter them.

Although following sustained relationships grief may persist for two years or more, there is life after bereavement and the vast majority of the bereaved, even the very elderly, come to reorganise and redirect their lives; involvement with outside agencies such as social clubs, local societies and Cruse (The National Organisation for the Widowed and their Children) may ease the transition to a new identity. Lapses into grief on special occasions — birthdays, Christmas, the anniversary of the death — may continue but become more manageable with the passage of time.

Cruse perhaps merits more discussion here. Founded in 1959, it now has more than 70 branches in Great Britain and, because of its nature, is able to stay involved with the bereaved after professionals have begun to reduce their input; there is practical help (for example, with the management of tax and finances) and social support. The organisation run an annual course on 'Counselling before and after bereavement' for all professionals who work with the dying and the bereaved; it has proved of great value to those undertaking it.

Members of the Primary Health Care Team must be aware of the atypical grief which may be seen in the elderly. Sometimes grief is inhibited, with little emotional response apparent; sometimes it becomes chronic, increasingly prolonged and intensified. Both situations require prompt recognition and treatment since severe depression, physical illness or premature death may ensue. Another group for whom special consideration is necessary comprise the offspring of elderly parents who may have cared for them to the end to the detriment of their own development. Rehabilitation following the death of the parent may be extraordinarily difficult, especially where employment cannot be found and the prospect of their own old age in lonely and reduced circumstances looms darkly ahead.

The last achievement

When the time comes, there is no greater service that the nurse can render to her elderly patient than the appropriate use of all her nursing skills to assist him in the achievement of a peaceful death. That service, however, makes great demands upon her, not only in terms of technical expertise, compassion and gentleness but also in terms of her total professional involvement in the dying process. Colin Murray Parkes[2] has written that 'terminal care is a matter of human relationships — it demands that we use the whole of ourselves to relate to our fellow human beings who are in trouble'. To watch and wait with families, to care and to grieve with them and yet to remain supportive and enabling requires of the nurse a personal acceptance of mortality and all that it implies, a maturity of outlook and approach. But we are all vulnerable and the caring load may be heavy and at times distressing; an understanding team from which to work, the opportunity to talk over feelings and anxieties with others, the confirmation that we are not alone in our strivings — these are all essential if, in sharing the patient's dying experience, the nurse is to help him realise 'the last achievement'.

References

1. Saunders, C., Care of the dying, *Nursing Times,* **72,** 1976. Quoted in Carver, V. and Liddiard, P. (editors), *An Ageing Population*, Open University Press, 1978
2. Parkes, C. M., Psychological aspects. In Saunders, C. M. S. (editor), *The Management of Terminal Illness,* Arnold, 1978

Further reading

Jury, M. and Jury, D., *Gramp,* Grossman, 1976 [depiction in words and photographs of a family's loving support for their dying grandfather]
Robbins, J. (editor), *Care of the Dying Patient and the Family,* Lippincott Nursing Series, Harper and Row, 1982
Collins, S. and Parker, E., *Essentials of Nursing: An Introduction*, Macmillan, 1987

Part 5   Conclusion: A Future for Old Age

Chapter 16   Towards the twenty-first century

Many readers will have heard the old story of the man who, stopped and asked for directions to a certain village, began, 'Well, of course, I wouldn't start from here . . .'. Given that, because of inadequate forward planning in the past, criticism is levelled against our current provision for elderly people as being largely 'crisis intervention', when looking to their future, perhaps we would not wish to start with what we have. Sir Ronald Gibson, Chairman of the Brendoncare Foundation, speaks of the British penchant for hit or miss types of care and for leaving things to the last moment; as earlier chapters indicated, many of our provisions developed more by accident than design, and we are left with areas of overlap, yawning gaps in services elsewhere and a growing, more demanding clientele whose needs are urgent. While acknowledging once more the point made in the first chapter of this book — the complete uniqueness of every individual — the remainder of this text seeks to put those needs more clearly into focus, with some broad suggestions as to how we as a caring society must proceed to meet them.

Implications for planning

> PAUSE FOR THOUGHT
>
> In earlier chapters we saw that our ageing population has an older profile than previously, and that it has a larger proportion of women than men, many of whom live alone. This elderly population is not evenly distributed throughout the country or within our towns and cities; it represents a relatively disadvantaged group of people.
> What are the implications of these features for:
>   (a) the elderly themselves?
>   (b) society generally?

Longfellow claimed that 'Age is opportunity no less than youth itself, though in another dress'; the first chapters of this book indicated how later life can be a positive, creative time for many people. But for old age to be such a time of growth and fulfilment, there would seem to be two definite prerequisites — satisfactory health and an adequate financial income. For a large number of older people these are not personal realities. In addition, the self-fulfilling prophecy syndrome, which has been described earlier, may — with society viewing the demographic changes as amounting to an 'elderly problem' rather than a challenge — see many older people having their negative expectations of old age reinforced.

But who better to challenge stereotypes and erroneous assumptions than elderly people themselves! Those now in their late middle years are perhaps the most active in local and national politics and in civic affairs; as the elderly of the future, by sheer weight of numbers, they will have greatly increased social and political clout and they must be prepared, demonstrating their contribution to society, to make their demands known in return. They must also be prepared actively to combat ageism and to exploit their potential to the full to better their lot. Although traditionally women have not taken a very active role politically, as the generations of women currently developing self-awareness and assertiveness age, it is hoped that the balance will be corrected. Often, however, the current generations of elderly women have developed quite considerably within their families the position of manager, leader and care giver; all of these attributes could be utilised now in political associations.

With regard to effective organising, elderly people in the UK could well take note of the Consultation of Older and Younger Adults (alias the Gray Panthers) in the United States, a movement dedicated to overcoming discrimination on the grounds of age and challenging the view that old, poor and stigmatised people are problems to society rather than the victims of it. They have made significant strides towards meeting their objectives under the charismatic leadership of Maggie Kuhn; appealing for choice and the right to self-determination in all aspects of life in old age, she once told a political gathering discussing the potential difficulties of later life: 'Give us the money you spend studying us and we can solve our own problems'.[1] The truth of her statement may well bear acting upon in our own British situation; equally important as increasing professional support systems in coming years will be projects to enable elderly people to help themselves. The active involvement of the young old in support of the older old has been discussed earlier; a survey in 1981 found 20% of the retired belonging to a voluntary organisation active in this capacity,[2] although many more assist friends and neighbours more informally.

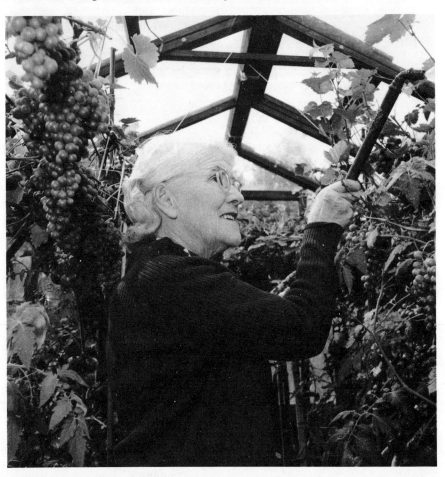

Society as a whole may have a variety of concerns about its elderly contingent, ranging from anxiety about the cost of their support to more altruistic considerations. The individuals making up that society, however, all have a vested personal interest in age and ageing, since the vast majority will personally experience the phenomenon — although in younger life they may well not wish to acknowledge the eventuality! Many will be required to act in a caring capacity, looking after elderly relatives or friends — and with changing work and social patterns, male carers may well increase in numbers too. There is an urgent need to recognise the importance of preparation for these phases of life, not only immediately before or at the time of their arrival, but also in a progressive fashion from much earlier years. Mention was made in Chapter 4 of preparation for retirement courses and the need for more concentration on women's issues; with the employment situation of the late twentieth century it could be that for some people there will be a need to prepare for a whole lifetime without paid employment, with emphasis on the constructive use of leisure and the gaining of recognition and a meaningful lifestyle in other ways. Whether transition to old age for these people will perhaps be less stressful remains to be seen.

How is an awareness of the reality of ageing to be stimulated in the general public? Changes in general educational input from childhood onwards are important; organisations such as Age Concern are very involved with school children and young people's groups. Emphasis is placed on the positive, constructive role of elderly people within a community as well as their special needs. There would now seem to be a greater appreciation of the dangers inherent in the use in fund raising appeals and the like of such lines as 'Old Mary is 86 and hardly ever leaves her cold room or talks to anyone . . .'. The assumptions implicit in such statements and similar media presentations adversely colour the expectations of those who from personal experience do not know better about age and ageing, and any guilt stimulated only rarely spurs useful action. A frequent response from the public when inadequacies in our system come to light is that 'something must be done about it' — the implication being that someone else (i.e. the State) should intervene. The message needs to be got across that as fellow human beings we all have a responsibility to 'do something about it' and that everyday neighbourliness is often more appropriate than a cascade of bureaucratic intervention.

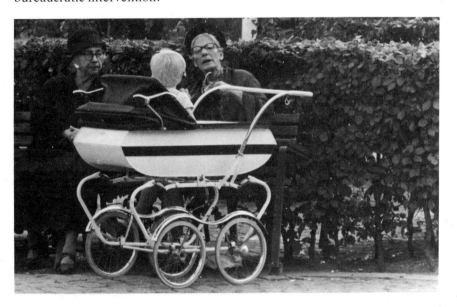

However, the State cannot escape its essential duties, and the creation of an environment suitable for an ageing population is crucial; account must be taken of older people's needs in housing, transport and shopping facilities, and in leisure and educational opportunities. Sadly, much lip service has been paid to these needs in the recent past and authorities may now feel that they have made suitable provision. In truth, many schemes have been designed and implemented without taking into account the express, informed wishes of the client group in question and are unimaginative and unattractive to them. For example, much sheltered housing has been developed away from everyday living facilities such as pubs and supermarkets, and residents may lead a ghetto type existence divorced from other age and social groups. Much of the basic environmental adaptation which would benefit older people would also be welcomed by other sectors of the community. Ramps rather than steps, wider doorways and more accessible public toilets would considerably help parents with young children in prams and pushchairs, for example, as well as older people with walking aids and wheelchairs.

Whatever provision is made for older people in the physical environment or in personal services, it needs to augment independence and not create dependence. This is important not only from the individual's point of view, but also because of the economic stringencies with which service providers are currently faced and which will continue certainly into the foreseeable future. Limited resources demand exceedingly careful allocation and accountability for professional action. National directives on allocation may not be appropriate, because of the geographical variation in the distribution of elderly people, as discussed above. Local needs must be carefully scrutinised and priorities set and acted upon; careful evaluation of service provision is mandatory to ensure that objectives are being met and that services continue to meet identified needs.

A major consideration in the coming decades will be to ensure an adequate financial income for our ageing population. More elderly people will be in receipt of pensions for longer periods of time and as they reach older old age will have additional health-related expenditure (for example, to meet heating and housing needs) which may stretch already limited incomes. Urgent examination of the situation and action is necessary to prevent twenty-first century pensioners having to experience the poverty their predecessors are living in now. Yet at the time of writing (Summer 1986) a new Social Security Bill is before the UK Parliament, the provisions of which many people feel will be detrimental to many already disadvantaged older people. It would seem that despite the Government's rhetoric there is little active commitment to positive action to improve the financial lot of elderly people.

The same could be seen to be true in relation to health and social services provision. Much has been spoken and written about the transfer of emphasis — and consequently of funds — to primary health care in the community from the prestigious hospital units (usually dominated by the medical establishment). At a time of limited resources it is only by such a shift that the necessary increased provision for elderly people can be made. Yet this, too, seems to be honoured more in the breach than in the observance. Even within specific geriatric units, where it might be expected that more enlightened attitudes would exist, there is often a concentration on more 'acute' types of care, with health promotional skills and the long-term needs of the frail elderly relatively overlooked. However, these are values neglected at our peril; there is ten times more spent on health and social service provision for those over 75 than for those between 15 and 65, and any avenue

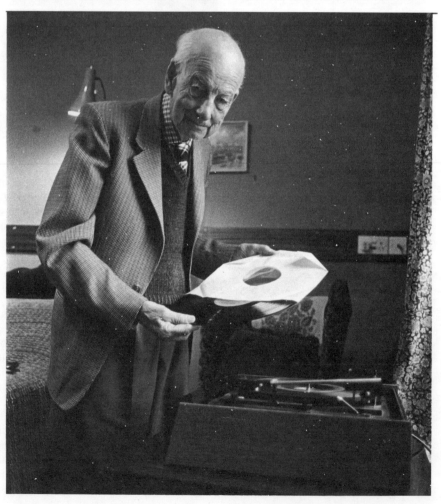

that could lead to a healthier, more active old age demands exploration. Preventive work is beneficial not only in terms of individual comfort and happiness, but also very much in cost-effective terms in the longer perspective.

As indicated in the Preface and illustrated throughout this book, health and social issues are inextricably linked for elderly people, with those in the poorest social circumstances faring considerably worse than the more privileged. Sadly, however, the 'powers that be' in health and social service provision do not share so strong a bond. Professionals come from very different backgrounds, have different emphases in their training, and often see situations very differently; they have very disparate financial systems and are not subject to any central coordination. Unless all those working with elderly people — in health care, local authorities, Department of the Environment, housing authorities and voluntary bodies — recognise that they are partners in caring, with no one group having the monopoly or all the answers, the fragmented approach which has dogged progress to date will simply continue.

Attention must also be given to the rift between State and private sectors. Understandably in those committed to the highest ideals of public service provision, feelings sometimes run high at the current increase in, and subsidised use of, independent facilities, but, with the projected increased needs, 'for the well-being of the frail aged, the public and private sectors must work together in a spirit of true cooperation combining the best each has to give'.[3]

Preparing nurses to meet future needs

In a book intended for nurses (both in training and trained) looking at the health needs of elderly people, it would seem appropriate to end by briefly considering the necessary preparation for professional practice to meet those needs in the future. At the time of writing nurses are discussing the proposals put forward by the United Kingdom Central Council in 'Project 2000 — A New Preparation for Practice', and it would seem that major changes in nurse education with far-reaching effects could be imminent.

To meet the needs of the future, the orientation of the nurse will certainly need to change, with far less emphasis put on illness and hospital care and far more on wellness and its promotion and on community involvement. Recognising that with elderly people especially families and friends are frequently the 'primary carers', it could well often be that the nurse, rather than being a direct giver of practical care, becomes a 'facilitator' for those informal carers, helping them to identify their needs and directing them towards resources available to meet them, advising and counselling. So much of our nurse education still concentrates on the 'doing for' aspects of caring; we need to stress and to develop the nurse's teaching role, her understanding of family and group dynamics. We need to increase her knowledge of neighbourhood organisations and other voluntary and statutory supports and to ensure that she becomes confident in and competent at referral procedures.

Mention has been made earlier of the new Nursing Home type units within the NHS. For the frail elderly for whom intensive community support is lacking or inadequate, ongoing care in such a nurse-managed environment is often appropriate; a further aspect of the nurse's role to be developed is that of worker in this style of provision. Traditional nursing approaches to care and ward management may be totally out of keeping with the philosophy underlying the development of such units, and careful preparation of students to promote a more democratic, flexible and creative manner will be required.

Research into aspects of nursing care of the elderly was also mentioned in earlier chapters. While forward strides in care have certainly been made in recent years, much of our work with older people still needs critical investigation and a consequent review of practices. To date, general nurse training has not truly stimulated an enquiring, open-minded approach — indeed it has often discouraged it. The chance to rectify this situation with a new type of nurse training must be seized now for the benefit of all our elderly patients.

A FINAL POINT TO PONDER

David Hobman, Director of Age Concern England, speaks of a caring society as one in which we are interested in an individual's potential rather than in limitations imposed by age or handicap.

What other changes in nurse education would help to make our profession a more caring society?

References

1. Kuhn, M., Speech delivered at Sangamon State University, Springfield, Illinois, April, 1975
2. *Growing Older,* Cmnd 8173, Chapter 4: Retirement, a time of opportunity; HMSO, 1981
3. Young, P., The public and private face of geriatric care, *British Journal of Geriatric Nursing,* March/April, 1986, 3

Further reading

All Our Tomorrows: Growing Old in Britain, Report of the BMA Board of Education and Science, 1986

Nuberg, C., *Programmes and Services for the Elderly in Industrialised Countries.* In Hobman, D. (editor), *The Impact of Ageing: Strategies for Care,* Croom Helm, 1981

Davies, A., Elderly, British and black, *Voluntary Action,* **13,** 1982, 18–19

Townsend, P. and Davidson, N. (editors), *Inequalities in Health; the Black Report,* Penguin Books, 1982

Index